PUT YOUR BRAIN FIRST

RADICALLY IMPROVE THE WAY YOU AGE

PUT YOUR BRAIN FIRST

RADICALLY IMPROVE THE WAY YOU AGE

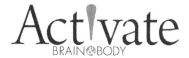

Niche Pressworks
INDIANAPOLIS, IN

PUT YOUR BRAIN FIRST

For permission to reprint portions of this content or bulk purchases,
contact info@activatebrainandbody.com

Published by Niche Pressworks; http://NichePressworks.com
Indianapolis, IN

ISBN: 978-1-952654-37-4 Paperback
       978-1-952654-38-1 eBook

TABLE OF CONTENTS

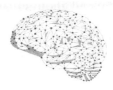

A COMPANY ON A MISSION

Activate Brain & Body is a brain health company.

We provide an innovative and completely new approach to brain and body health by combining breakthroughs in neuroscience with the latest findings on brain and body fitness physiology—all targeting advances in longevity. The result? An approach tailored to meet the needs of an aging population looking for solutions. People who are asking: Can my brain last as long as my body? Can I defy aging and stay active and sharp into my 90s and perhaps beyond?

Our inspiration came from looking at trends over the past decade. We've noted an aging population, rapidly rising healthcare costs, concerns about declining health with longer lifespans, and increased concerns about cognitive decline, dementia, and Alzheimer's. These are worrisome prospects and part of what inspired us to write this book. We know we can be a part of the solution and make a difference.

Research clearly supports that certain types of physical and cognitive exercise build brain health.

After years of research, development, and trial programs, it has all come together under one roof by a group of people united around a mission: **to radically improve the trajectory of aging and to operationalize what we have learned about creating brain fitness.**

We believe Activate Brain & Body can help people live happier, healthier, and longer lives. Our approach can give them the independence to do whatever they desire, whether that's continuing to work productively, enjoying sports or travel, or spending time with great-grandchildren.

Activate Brain & Body can also reduce your healthcare costs by slowing, minimizing, or preventing the conditions that shorten your health span: cognitive decline, dementia, metabolic syndrome, and more. Our approach empowers people to ignore the indignities of aging and remain active, sharp, independent, and vital.

And the best news of all is that when you focus on building better brain health, you also build a much better body. That's why we say "Put Your Brain First"...because your body will follow.

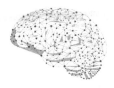

CHAPTER 1

IS AGING INEVITABLE?

Age is no barrier; it's a limitation you put on your mind.
—JACKIE JOYNER-KERSEE

"Look younger overnight!"
"Feel like your old self again."
"Take 20 years off your age in only 15 minutes a day!"

If headlines like these have caught your eye, you're not alone. Our society is obsessed with aging—or rather, NOT aging. In fact, in 2020 alone, an estimated $58.5 billion was spent on anti-aging efforts worldwide, and that doesn't account for money spent on healthcare or fitness.[1]

But the results of these efforts are often only skin-deep, at least when it comes to alleviating our real worries about the years to come. While our complexion might look a little dewier and our hair may be a little less grey, we're still preoccupied with concerns about the future.

Will Our Brains Last as Long as Our Bodies?

Can we avoid the indignities that aging often brings? Will we be able to maintain the quality of life we dream of? Is how we age entirely a matter of genetics? Is there something we can do to extend not only the number of our years but also the quality of those years?

As you'll learn throughout this book, Activate team members were asking these same questions and had very personal reasons for wanting to create a simple, functional approach to life-long fitness of brain and body.

We began our quest ten years ago by scouring the research on aging, neuroscience, fitness, nutrition, and stress management. As we began to formulate a program, we tested our theories out with groups of men and women aged 45 plus. To our absolute delight and gratification, our predictions were proven true and further validated by rigorous academic and medical research.

After numerous discussions with people who shared their worries with us as well as our own experiences with aging relatives, the team at Activate Brain & Body tasked ourselves with answering one question:

> **Is aging inevitable?**
> The answer is...yes. Getting chronologically older is an inescapable reality. But the steep cognitive and physical decline that so many people experience in later years is NOT inevitable. *You can indeed take charge of the way you age.*

We were determined to find a way that forward-thinking individuals, even those with family members who have experienced cognitive and/or physical decline, could delay the loss of cognitive or physical function that can come with age, so they could remain independent, healthy, and happy longer.

Here's the great news: There are specific behaviors, habits, and actions that anyone can take to increase the ability to live a longer, happier, healthier life in both body and brain. It is possible to offset or delay the indignities of aging and live an active, full, happy life until your final days. It is possible to both prolong your life and increase your quality of life. We may not be able to AVOID aging, but we can REDEFINE aging.

But before we jump into exactly what the solution is, let's take a look at two people, Sharon and Darwin.

A Tale of Two Futures

While it seems like we're bombarded almost daily with promises for entering our 50s, 60s, 70s, and beyond with youthful skin and the abs of a 30-year-old, we have also seen far too many of our parents and older relatives and friends age in brain and body well before their time—like Sharon.

We all know someone like Sharon, a vivacious, lively mother and grandmother who spent a lifetime building a family and mentoring young people as a professional educator. Then, in her early 60s, her family started to notice slight changes.

A forgotten name. A missed appointment. A lapse in memory that, unfortunately, pointed to a bigger issue: Alzheimer's.

Quickly—much too quickly—her decline became so severe that her husband of almost 50 years was unable to care for her at home.

Now she resides in a memory care facility. It's a lovely place, and her family visits regularly, but she rarely recognizes them. The joyful retirement years she and her husband had dreamed of have vanished, consumed by a fog of hazy memories and half-forgotten faces.

She and her family have been robbed of years of connection, laughter, and experiences—a theft that is all too familiar to many people with aging parents. This family also shares with millions of others the now-familiar questions they invariably ask in retrospect:

- What could we have done differently years earlier to offset or delay the cognitive decline?

- What lifestyle changes could we all have implemented to postpone or prevent this from happening?

- What things can I do now to not share a similar fate?

Now, let's meet Darwin.

Raised during the Depression, Darwin has continuously stayed active mentally and physically. A lawyer by profession, he has always lifted weights or played with some sort of strengthening device even while watching TV. Likewise, he has a lifelong love affair with new experiences, bonding instantly with anyone who shares his passion for golf and traveling extensively in his younger years.

Now 90, Darwin is still extremely curious, spending hours online exploring topics such as psychology, automobiles, and politics, as well as playing online bridge. He walks daily for at least a mile, still drives, does daily exercises with weights, engages with neighbors and strangers alike, and offers legal advice.

Darwin now lives with his daughter but maintains his independence. He makes his own meals, drives, handles his medical appointments, balances his checkbook, does his own shopping, and manages his medications.

While he's experiencing some physical and cognitive decline, he's well above expectations for his age. He seems to have mastered the art of aging well.

For years, the Activate founders have been looking to science for ways to help people add more health and function to their brain and body years. We wanted to identify specific actions that contributed to Darwin's high physical and cognitive function in his 90s and identify actions that might have helped Sharon in her 60s. We wanted to determine if it would be possible to help people of all ages take charge of the way they age.

Specifically, why do some individuals move into their later years retaining their mental edge and physical ability, while others are struck with debilitating cognitive issues, even though they were physically in good shape? Was it genetics or something more? And if so, what?

These questions and the topic of aging led us to the fitness industry for answers. Unfortunately, this 96 billion dollar powerhouse is part of the problem.[2]

The Traditional Fitness Industry Ignores Brain Health

The fitness industry misses the mark on a few important points. First, it views the brain and body as separate mechanisms. Despite being part of the same entity, exercise programs typically separate the brain and body. Second, traditional fitness centers and gyms often ignore the unique needs of the aging population.

Together, these two missteps have contributed to a health crisis—a whole generation that has spent an average of 20 percent of their total years in poor physical or cognitive condition.[3]

These observations made us wonder how the fitness industry could have gotten things so wrong. One of the main things we noted was that the majority of fitness facilities are designed for and marketed to twenty- to thirty-somethings. These younger people are typically interested in perfecting their physique or training for athletic endeavors. In fact, many of these fitness facilities pitch the latest trends in fitness, extreme cardio, fad diets, and a one-size-fits-all approach rather than personalized plans that improve functional fitness and maintain cognitive levels. These objectives make it seem like much of the traditional fitness industry forgets that anyone over 50 even exists.

Focusing only on the physical aspects of fitness neglects the cognitive benefits of exercise, a critical element that we will delve into throughout this book (and that we have developed in our trial and research, such as The Cognitive Circuit™. It also means that many people who could benefit from a program that combines physical exercise with cognitive challenges are unlikely to find a home anywhere in the existing fitness industry.

Opting out of fitness clubs by choosing to work out at home isn't a great solution either. It can be expensive, tedious, lonely, and downright boring. Even the latest online apps and videos have their limitations. They often lack personalized workout solutions, which makes it harder to exercise with correct form and can result in injuries.

Because many people above age 45 do not feel welcome at the gym and home options are less than optimal, many people end up doing nothing at all. Lack of motivation, lack of structure, and lack of knowledge all contribute to inertia, meaning that each year, people become a little less fit, a little less limber, and a little less strong.

On top of that, even people who embrace physical fitness as a lifestyle aren't safe from the cognitive decline that leads to a deteriorating brain in a functioning body. Many of us have seen aging friends and family members who, despite their active lives, end up unable to care for themselves.

So what can you do?

Transforming Research Into Action

Luckily, this is an exciting time to be in the fitness field. Many recent discoveries in neurology, neuroscience, kinesiology, fitness, and nutrition outline specific actions people can take to keep their brains sharp and illuminate the link between a healthy brain and body.

Most importantly, the science shows that you can take charge of the way you age.

The challenge then becomes how to apply these new scientific findings to create a workable fitness plan. The vast amount of information and opinions can feel confusing. Self-proclaimed experts, television doctors, women's magazines, the lady at the health food store, and even Uber drivers all have opinions on what we can do to protect our brain and body against aging.

Unfortunately, there's no guarantee that the information they're passing on is accurate or even safe. Your aunt, for instance, might tell you to eat six almonds a day to improve your memory because she took one element of a much larger study out of context, simply not understanding the bigger picture.

One of the main challenges for those on a quest for lifelong health is determining what is science and what is pure science fiction. If you don't have a degree in nutrition, kinesiology, or neuroscience (or all three), it can be difficult to decode the science. Not only can the information be tough to understand, but also it often seems to contradict itself.

That's where Activate can help. Our team of experts includes certified brain health trainers, certified functional fitness trainers, a clinical psychologist, and PhDs in kinesiology and exercise science. We are uniquely qualified to connect the dots and create individualized plans based on what the science tells us. At Activate Brain & Body, we transform the science and data into realistic and achievable plans that will help you redefine aging.

By simplifying the process of staying fit and ensuring your brain lasts as long as your body, you can spend more of your years as active, independent, strong, and vital as you desire. We can empower *you* to take control of the way you age.

The Bottom Line

The bottom line is that certain types of exercise, combined with specific cognitive training techniques, capitalize on the brain's ability to restructure and strengthen itself against decline.

What's more, when we focused our training on brain-health-building activities first, improvements to our participants' bodies followed! This discovery was huge.

> Our results showed that it is possible to build a sharper, more resilient brain. Even better, when you do so using the Activate process, all measures of physiological fitness—cardiac health, reaction times, agility and balance, endurance—also improve.

The Activate team now had evidence that only by putting brain health *first* could the full benefits of current cognitive health discoveries be put into practice.

Our next step involved creating a simple structure for sharing our findings with 50 percent of the population (the percentage of adults over age 50 in the US). No doubt, all of these adults want to live independent, meaningful lives while enjoying cognitive and physical health.

At Activate, we reject the common wisdom that steep cognitive and physical decline is inevitable. Instead, we know that you can live an active, full, happy, and independent life into your 80s, 90s, and beyond...like our friend Darwin. We know there are many more Darwins out there who are looking for solutions on their quest for a happier, healthier, longer life.

A Public Mission with Personal Roots

Rare is the American who can reach the age of 50 without knowing—or being related to—someone who had aged poorly, and our team at Activate is no exception. We've watched as friends and loved ones experienced the painful consequences of severe cognitive deterioration, such as Alzheimer's. Seeing a formerly active and sharp individual slowly slip away is nothing short of excruciating, as Sharon's family can attest.

Sharon isn't a made-up example, though her story is familiar to many. She's actually a real person, the mother of one of the Activate founders, Rex Bevis. And Darwin isn't a figment of our imagination, either; he's the father of another Activate founder, Alison Kal, who recently lost her mother to dementia.

Alison and Rex are not alone in feeling a personal connection with the goals of Activate Brain & Body. The entire team believes deeply in our mission, and that's what drives us all: the desire to radically improve what individuals across the country and around the world will experience as they age.

We've done the hard part for you. We've done the research, tested the approach, refined the process, and figured out what actually moves the needle when it comes to improving the functioning of your brain and body, for today, for tomorrow, and for the future.

Keep reading, and we'll show you how you can take advantage of this new approach to brain-body fitness. Your independent and strong future self will thank you!

Try This Assessment

Does this sound like you? Check all that apply:

☐ I have a family history of dementia or Alzheimer's.

☐ Sometimes a word or name is on the tip of my tongue, and it takes me a minute to recall it.

☐ I don't feel comfortable in a traditional fitness club.

☐ I sit too much, and I move too little.

☐ I find myself forgetting why I walked into a room.

☐ I find myself driving at slower speeds or reacting more slowly when I drive.

☐ I have trouble remembering someone's name immediately after I meet them.

☐ I have not taken up a new sport or physical activity in the last three years.

☐ I have been diagnosed with high cholesterol, high blood pressure, and/or diabetes.

☐ I prefer to keep to the familiar in my day-to-day life, and I am uncomfortable stepping outside my normal routine or environment.

If you've checked some of these boxes, read on and learn why you should consider taking action to take charge of the way you are aging.

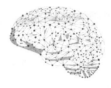

CHAPTER 2

YOU CAN TAKE CHARGE
OF THE WAY YOU AGE

If I knew I was going to live this long, I would
have taken better care of myself.
—MICKEY MANTLE

Baseball Hall of Famer Mickey Mantle believed his future health was hard-coded into his genes. For most of his life, he believed he would inevitably fall victim to Hodgkin's lymphoma at a young age, as his father and grandfather had done.

Resigned to a shortened lifespan, he resolved to live the years he had to the fullest with little concern for how his actions would impact an old age he never planned to see. It wasn't until his 60s that he realized his poor lifestyle choices had shortened his life. He died of complications from injury and alcohol abuse—not Hodgkin's—at age 63.

Even just a generation or two ago, Mantle's *que será, será* attitude was not uncommon. People largely believed that genetics was destiny; if your parents died young, you would, too. There was little you could do to move the needle one way or the other, as the die had already been cast. So if you were to make it to the big 6-0, you'd better slow down, take it easy, and enjoy the few years you had left.

Our thinking has taken a hard turn for the better in the last decade. We now know genetics isn't irrefutable. Not only can your life last well beyond 60, but you can also live well in your later years. Thanks to scientific research, healthcare, medical and surgical advances, and better lifestyle choices, today's adults in midlife and beyond are changing the very meaning of what it is to grow older. And it all starts in the brain, as we'll see later in this chapter.

What Is "Old"?

Ask a five-year-old what is "old," and she'll say, "Mommy and Daddy"—even if Mommy and Daddy are in their 20s!

Ask a 50-year-old what is considered "old," and she'll say the same thing, but this time Mommy and Daddy are in their 70s.

And ask a boomer what is considered "old," and she'll point at her neighbor in his 80s or 90s.

Humans have an interesting ability to adjust our perspective on life, depending on where we're standing. And as our culture shifts, so does the concept of what's universally considered to be "old age."

According to the American Society of Gerontologists:

- 45 to 64 is middle age.
- 65 to 74 is young-old.

- 75 to 84 is categorized as old.
- 85 to 94 is categorized as old-old.
- 95-plus is called oldest old (and the fastest-growing age group of all).

Contrast these categories to 1920 when US life expectancy was 59 years—what we'd now consider firmly in the middle years![4] We not only expect to live longer, but we also expect our kids to push the edges of longevity even farther than we have.

Almost 50 million people in the United States are over 65, according to the 2016 census, and 20.6 million of those are over 75.[5] In 2045, the first of the baby boomers will turn 100. Given current life expectancy rates, there are going to be a good number of centenarians (actually the fastest-growing age cohort on a percentage basis).

These aging boomers will continue to shape culture and the country as we enter the post-pandemic years after 2020. This group has already begun redefining what it means to age.

For instance, the Boston Consulting Group estimates that by 2030, the 55-plus population in the US will have accounted for half of all domestic consumer spending growth since the global financial crisis of 2008, with the numbers even higher overseas.[6]

People above age 50 are driving a huge portion of the world's economic activity, which means more resources and attention will be spent to address longevity issues like physical health, cognitive health, quality of life, financial planning, and more. More people are getting older, but that doesn't mean you have to feel—or act—old.

Change Your Thinking: You're Not Old

We've all heard that age is just a number, and you're only as old as you feel. There's truth to that statement. Research has shown that by thinking younger, your body can actually reverse its aging.

Ellen Langer, a Harvard psychologist, believed that "Wherever you put the mind, you're necessarily putting the body."[7] Her theory was that if you surrounded older people with reminders of their younger years, they'd start acting—and feeling—younger. She and her grad students constructed an immersive experience in which their participants—eight men in their 70s—would be transported back in time to 1959 for a week.

Everything about the retreat was set up to recreate 1959—from the music to the food to the magazines and books on the shelves. Participants were told to act as if it were 1959, discussing events as if they were happening in real time. Langer details in her book *Counterclockwise* how the men's physical strength, dexterity, posture, memory, hearing, and more had improved just by the end of the week.

Her hypothesis had been proven: How you think changes how you feel and act. The team at Activate has taken that adage a step farther: You can feel younger and defy aging by being active in both brain and body.

Becca Levy's research further supports this brain-body connection. Her work at the Yale School of Public Health has shown that shifting your mindset can add years to your life. In other words, positive thinking pays off—to the tune of as much as seven years of added lifespan, even if you start in midlife.[8]

According to the American Society of Gerontologists, we aren't considered "old" until we're over 75. So, we're going to be blunt: If you're under 75, you're simply not old by today's standards, so stop referring to yourself that way. And if you're over 75? Well, there's still a lot you can do to change the trajectory of how you age by thinking, living, appearing, and acting much younger, so you're not really old either!

We want to emphasize one important point: Research on aging and how we can change how we age is constantly being updated and discovered. New approaches to everything from nutrition to pharmaceuticals to biomechanics are evolving, and the effects are being felt across industries as diverse as healthcare and technology.

You might be wondering, "What if I wasn't in that great a shape even in my younger years? Is it too late now?" Great news: Even if you weren't fit in your 40s or 50s, you can still benefit by improving your brain and body in your 60s and 70s. As Dr. Levy's research shows, it's never too late to start. Any efforts you make today will pay off tomorrow and into the future—which hopefully will be a long one!

The Life in Your Years, Not the Years in Your Life

Though we all want to live longer, we're equally concerned about how we live. We're not content to live out the last decades in decline or in a wheelchair, confined in body and mind. Quality of life matters, and we want both length and depth to our years.

Take a look at the following chart:

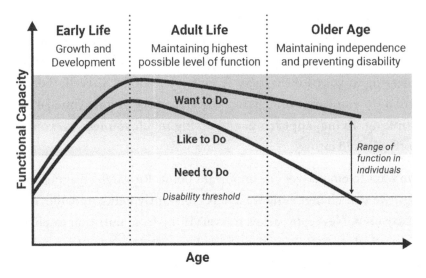

Figure 1: Functional capacity over time. You can raise
the curve. You can change the way you age.

Chart credit: Functional Aging Institute.

For most of us, the goal is to avoid falling below the "disability threshold," the place where our function has dropped to the point where we are no longer able to care for ourselves.

If that occurs, we can't cook for ourselves or care for our own personal hygiene needs, let alone take a trip to Hawaii or enjoy an afternoon at the park with the grandkids. Our mental functions have also declined, leaving us dependent, inactive, and likely depressed.

If we fall below the "disability threshold," we're bedridden, or nearly so, with a severe limit on how we can interact with and enjoy life. We're spending large sums on caretakers, assisted living homes, medications, therapies, and other interventions that have little if any effect in returning us to normalcy.

The worst-case, end-of-life scenario is a long, slow, complicated, painful, and expensive decline. In 2018, Americans spent $3.65 trillion on health care. Ten percent, or $365 billion of it, went for end-of-life care.[9]

A much better alternative—and one that we at Activate Brain & Body believe is quite attainable—is a long, active, healthy life and then a brief amount of time in decline as we approach our last days. This has become known as "compressed morbidity," and it is a desirable goal for many. With compressed morbidity, you avoid the long, slow, medically expensive, and emotionally distressing decline to death. Instead, you "live long, die fast."

While no program can guarantee longevity, treating brain and body fitness as preventive medicine provides a best-case scenario, giving you the mental and physical reserves to draw from in your later years.

The fact is, you can take charge of the way you age by choosing to be fit in both brain and body. That choice—and the subsequent behaviors you adopt—can change the trajectory of your aging.

Forget about that long, slow, medically expensive decline into inactivity, illness, and dependency. Instead, choose a path that allows you to live longer, enjoy your days, see your great-grandchildren, be more productive, and have more fun. Choose to be fit until the end.

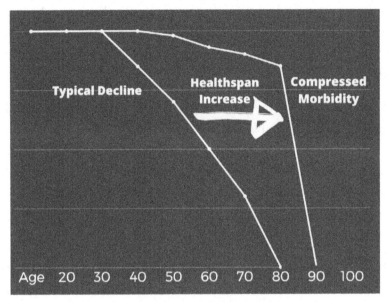

Figure 2: Compressed morbidity creates a much
longer health span. Live long, die fast.

Aging Differently

It's impossible to talk about longevity without talking about finances.
As we addressed earlier in this chapter, getting older can cost you
big—even if you stay healthy until the end.

Looking at a longer life forces you to ask yourself the hard questions:
Will my retirement fund run out before I do? Will declining health
bankrupt me or force my family to care for me? Can I even afford to
retire? What will I do with myself after I retire? Ensuring that you
have enough financial assets to fund your lifestyle at the level you
desire may mean you delay retirement, by necessity or by choice.

People, in general, are working longer. It used to be that 55 was the
standard retirement age; now, the average retirement age is 64, with
many people working longer.[10]

Not only are people pushing off retirement, but they're also wondering why they'd even want to! At 64 years old, you've likely got decades left. What are you going to do with those remaining years? Play bingo? Binge-watch Netflix…for ten hours a day?

At Activate Brain & Body, we see that a key part of longevity and increased health span is the freedom to work. Working brings rewards beyond financial, including a sense of purpose, social connection, and even increased lifespan.[11]

We're determined to help you live the life you want to live as long as you can. And to achieve that goal, we view aging differently—not as something to avoid but as a reality of life that can be impacted and enhanced. We do that by viewing brain and body fitness as preventive healthcare.

> By investing in yourself now, you may be able to significantly reduce the need for medical intervention, drugs, and many healthcare services in your later years. That can happen when you put your brain first.

Brain Before Body

Fitness goals shift as we age. We become less concerned with achieving washboard abs or looking like a 30-year-old movie celebrity or Olympic athlete—if that ever was our aim. Instead, our focus shifts to maintaining function.

Instead of wondering how much we can deadlift or how fast we can run a 10K, we're thinking:

- Can I fend off cognitive decline and stay sharp?

- Will my vision and reaction speed and processing speed stay sharp enough to continue to drive safely?

- Do I have the stamina to take that hiking trip to the Grand Canyon?

- Can I keep up with my grandkids or great grandkids at Disney World?

- Can I live a happier, healthier, longer life and live independently without needing an in-home aide or full-time care?

- What can I do now to stave off the functional decline of my brain and body to prevent poor quality of life in my 80s and 90s?

While many of these questions deal with physical health and fitness, we've learned that everything—including physical parameters—actually starts in the brain. The more we focus on improving cognitive function, the more the entire body will benefit.

Here's a great example of how brain function oversees body function. We've all heard of muscle memory, right? Basically, you repeat a specific motor task or movement until it is committed to memory. But muscle memory is a fallacy. Your muscles cannot think!

What we've been calling muscle memory actually involves strands of interconnected brain cells aligning to control complex movements: these neural pathways guide the muscles that make you move. It's always been all about the brain.

So it makes sense that the more we focus on improving brain function, the more the whole body will benefit. That's why we put the brain first, and the science of that is what we cover in the next chapter.

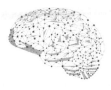

CHAPTER 3

WHY WE PUT THE BRAIN FIRST

The chief function of the body is to carry the brain around.
—THOMAS A. EDISON

You've likely heard the advice to create a financial "rainy day fund." This designated amount of money is set aside as protection against an uncertain future. While things may be humming along just fine in the present, we know all too well that roofs leak, cars break down, people get sick, and jobs disappear. Having a cushion—a financial reserve—can help insulate us against the ups and downs of fate.

What if we could do the same thing with our brains and our bodies? What if there were a way to store backup capacity for the future, so we have reserves to draw upon when needed?

While this concept may have been a pipe dream in previous generations, significant breakthroughs have occurred in the area of brain health that have led to the understanding that it is actually possible to delay the loss of function of our brains and bodies that normally comes with aging.

As we age, our brains shrink as neurons die. This brain shrinkage triggers a functional decline in both processing speed (how long it takes the brain to process and react to information—a skill critical for driving) and working memory (the ability to hold, manipulate, process, and store information—such as recalling people's names and occupations).

Studies have shown that the effects of aging on the brain can be decelerated by engaging in certain activities that can cause structural changes in the brain and create backup pathways or cognitive reserve.[12]

Likewise, our bodies change as we age—if you couldn't already tell! For example, without intervention, muscle strength for most adults peaks between 20 and 30. After that, strength slowly declines, eventually resulting in telling symptoms of muscle weakness, such as falling and difficulty with essential daily tasks–lifting heavy items out of your SUV, playing your favorite sport, climbing many flights of stairs, or running with the grandkid. However, the decline can be minimized or even offset by maintaining or creating the proper physical reserves (the excess capacity your body possesses to accomplish physical tasks, which decrease with age).

In this chapter, we'll dive into what we now know about the brain and how Activate has incorporated the latest research in brain health into our program to benefit both brain and body.

The Nun "Escapees"

Our knowledge about brain health increased exponentially in the 1990s as a result of the publication of what is widely referred to as "the

Nun Study," funded by the National Institute on Aging. By tracking almost 700 nuns in their 70s, the study aimed to identify what activities or experiences might have an impact on cognitive, neurological, and physical abilities over time.

One of the most remarkable discoveries was the result of individuals, such as Sister Bernadette, whose brain autopsies after death showed evidence of Alzheimer's but whose cognitive performance had remained above average throughout their lives. A link was established between the participants who were most cognitively and physically active during their lives and the retention of cognitive performance.

Yakov Stern, a researcher at Columbia University, coined the term cognitive reserve to explain how some people cope and function better than others with the same amount of damage to the brain. Here are the critical takeaways:

1. It is possible to build cognitive reserve through specific lifestyle activities.

2. It's never too late to add to your store of cognitive reserve.

Additional research suggests that as many as 25 percent of elderly adults, like Sister Bernadette, are "escapees" who appear cognitively intact while their brains at autopsy actually showed changes in brain tissue associated with Alzheimer's. These findings launched research aimed at figuring out how some individuals "escape" cognitive decline (despite showing physiological aspects of it) and how that outcome can be replicated by other aging adults.

The Myth of the Fixed Brain

To understand how Sister Bernadette and others were able to escape the symptoms of Alzheimer's, we have to tackle a myth about the human brain. Quite simply, you are NOT born with a finite number of neurons (brain cells). New neurons are created throughout your life, especially in the hypothalamus, which is your memory center.

But it's not enough to merely generate new brain cells. In order for your brain to derive the benefit of this neurogenesis and for these new neurons to thrive, two conditions typically occur.

First, the new neurons get nourished with brain-derived neurotrophic factor, or BDNF, a hormone your body naturally generates by physical exercise. BDNF is sometimes referred to as Miracle-Gro® for the brain because it improves the function of neurons, encourages new neurons to grow, and protects them from stress and cell death. Aerobic exercise not only generates BDNF but also supports the growth of new blood vessels in the brain.

Second, new neurons must find a way to connect with other neurons to form networks, a process called neuroplasticity. In other words, your brain changes over time. It is not a closed system with a set number of elements that behave in set manners. Instead, new, stimulating experiences (such as learning ballroom dancing, perfecting your tennis serve, jumping rope, and many other activities) literally excite the network and make the connections between neurons stronger and more prevalent.

Conversely, neural networks that are not used will grow weaker. Think about trying to recall the layout of streets in a town in which you once lived but no longer visit; over time, it becomes harder and harder to recall if Elm Street comes before or after Main Street and if the big church is at the corner of South and Broad or South and Bell. Use it or lose it is so true with the brain!

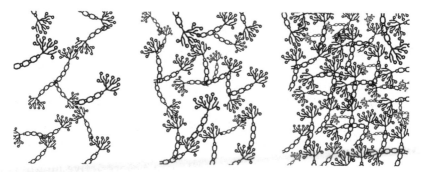

Figure 3. L to R: Building denser neural networks and cognitive reserve

There is strong evidence that the brain changes its very structure with every experience, adapting and perfecting circuits to become more efficient. This process, which begins in the womb, will not cease until the day you die. Whatever your age, how you live your life and the activities you choose literally change your brain. And if you want to increase neuroplasticity and strengthen your neural networks, you've got to move your body.

Building Cognitive Reserve

When you visit an Activate Brain & Body center, it's no accident that you'll find our facilities resemble an upscale fitness center. That's because the number one most documented—and most powerful— driver of neuroplasticity and cognitive reserve is physical activity.

This might be puzzling at first. After all, for years, we've been told by the experts to do Sudoku or a daily crossword puzzle to keep our brains sharp. Now, though, scientists have discovered that it's actually the body that supports brain health. Regular physical activity improves brain function in two ways. The physical movement boosts blood flow to the brain and stimulates the creation of the nerve growth factors and hormones involved in neurogenesis and neuroplasticity. These structural and functional changes are most notable in the parts of the brain typically associated with declines related to aging and cognitive impairment.

We've already discussed how aerobic exercise supports brain health with the release of BDNF. To further explain why physical activity supports expanded brain function, we need to go back two million years. At this point in time, the human species was transitioning from relatively sedentary forest dwellers to a more active hunting and gathering existence.

This new lifestyle paired high levels of physical activity with increased cognitive demands for motor control, memory, spatial navigation, and executive functions. All of these skills helped early humans track and kill woolly mammoths while scouring the surrounding countryside for edible berries and fungi. Our ancestors evolved to be running thinkers, and increased brain capacity was paired with increased physical activity—a connection that still holds today.

Resistance, or strength training, has been shown to activate an additional growth hormone, IGF-1. IGF-1 helps neurons differentiate and survive and also supports executive function and working memory. The dynamic duo of BDNF from aerobic exercise and IGF-1 from strength training provides a neurochemical "bath," helping neurons attach to networks.

Physical activity isn't the only way to spark neuroplasticity. As the descendants of runners who think and decide, our brains are also primed to respond to new and different (particularly cognitively) challenging activities.

Large group studies have shown improvements in attention, processing speed, memory, and even driving skills and safety as a result of cognitive training interventions such as specific computerized brain games. Brain scans of participants have shown an increase in white matter, which is the wiring between neurons. More white matter means stronger network connections and better brain health.

Don't Forget the Body

We've spoken in earlier chapters about our desire to maintain both brain and body function as we age. To avoid having a sharp brain in a declining body, physical reserve is also something to think about.

It's a great two-for-one system. Physical activity helps build cognitive reserve and is also a critical aspect of physical reserve. Strength training, in particular, is essential to offset the three to five percent of muscle strength we start to lose each decade beginning in our 30s.

> As Robert Butler of the National Institute on Aging says, "If exercise could be packaged in a pill, it would be the single most widely prescribed and beneficial medicine in the nation."

In fact, studies consistently show that a combination of both physical and cognitive exercise is what most effectively impacts how we age. Physical exercise encourages neuroplasticity, while cognitive exercise guides the new neurons into networks. Clinical trials show that combining the two in what's called dual-task training produces better results. In fact, physical and cognitive improvements occur more quickly with this approach than when just one approach is used.

That's why the centerpiece of the Activate Brain & Body program is The Cognitive Circuit™, an innovative and personalized program that guides members to the optimal conditions for building cognitive reserve. We'll dive more into The Cognitive Circuit™ in chapter 6.

Summing It Up

You can't stop the aging process, but you can exert control over how well you age. The difference between "escapees" like Sister Bernadette and those who age poorly all comes down to the presence of physical and cognitive reserves.

You can think of these reserves as two rainy-day savings accounts. Until midlife, you're automatically making direct deposits into your accounts. As you age, you'll need to make withdrawals, which will be small at first but will get larger over time. The key is to keep your balance in the green. And that's where The Cognitive Circuit™ comes into play.

The Cognitive Circuit™ is designed to help you continue to make deposits into your physical and cognitive reserve accounts even as the normal aging process makes withdrawals, ensuring you always have enough to maintain a positive balance.

Now that you know why cognitive and physical reserves are so crucial, let's talk about how to start making deposits into your accounts.

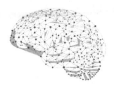

CHAPTER 4

EASY FIRST STEPS TO BRAIN HEALTH

The journey of a thousand miles begins with one step.
—LAO TZU

By now, you've hopefully started to get a glimmer of why the Activate Brain & Body team is so excited about the latest developments and research regarding creating cognitive and physical reserves. Aging doesn't have to look like what it was 50, 20, or even 10 years ago. We now have the ability to create a different kind of future, one that assumes a healthy brain and a healthy body.

You might be wondering, though, how to get started. The research is significant and convincing, but how do you translate the latest scientific findings into easy actions you can implement in your everyday life? That's what this chapter is about. It provides a beginner's guide to taking your first steps toward creating a lifestyle that supports brain health. In the upcoming pages, you'll see just how easy it is to get started!

Before you begin, however: get a physical. If you've been inactive or have any concerns about your ability to walk or exercise, please see a physician before you start. You want to make sure your heart and cardiovascular system are not compromised; your ankles, knees, and hips can take the strain; and your balance is fine. Once you're cleared, your doctor should celebrate your desire to get fit in this manner.

Next, **if you smoke, quit.** Right now. Just do it. Quitting smoking is the best thing you can do to prevent a long list of potential maladies from occurring. The perfect time to do it is when you begin a program for brain health. Your entire body will thank you, and you'll really benefit from the extra lung power you get by quitting. We know how hard it is to become a nonsmoker, and our coaches can address this within your individualized Activate Program.

Also, get a fitness tracker. This is something we feel pretty strongly about. Fitness tracking devices are part of what's called the Quantified Self movement, which simply means using devices to track biometric and movement information. These devices are incredibly useful — Fitbit®, Myzone®, Garmin®, Polar®, Suunto, Apple Watch®, and more. Take your pick. They are all good first steps. (When you join Activate, you'll get a Myzone device, but we'll get to that later on).

Measuring your physical activity makes a big difference. It's easy to measure your progress by comparing workouts across time. Tracking that progress (in steps, distance, calories burned, flights climbed, etc.) is both motivational and fun. That's just for starters.

As you progress, you're also going to want to carefully measure your heart rate because a key element in a healthier brain and body is getting your heart rate elevated enough to trigger real physiological improvement.

Why Brain Health?

As you've seen in previous chapters, brain health is the critical foundation upon which we can build cognitive and physical reserves. Brain health refers to your ability to effectively manage your daily life at work and at home. From making decisions to problem-solving to relational and communication components, a healthy brain lays the framework for an active and healthy life.

Revisiting the chart from chapter 2 on functional capacity, it's clear that over time, we naturally lose cognitive and physical function—but not all of us see the same level of decline. The difference in range of function between individuals, as indicated by the two arcs, can be attributed, in part, to the differing levels of cognitive reserve.

Cognitive reserve helps keep us "in the black," staving off age-related cognitive decline by providing backup capacity to support our brain performance. Cognitive reserve helps support brain health by compensating for the brain shrinkage that normally starts around midlife—even before we're aware of any symptoms. If not kept in check, it can lead to a decline below the disability threshold.

Here's a refresher on just some of what we now know about brain health and cognitive reserve:

You CAN generate new brain cells. We used to think brain cells couldn't regenerate, but scientists have confirmed that the brain can generate new cells at any age through a process called neurogenesis.

It's a natural process that happens throughout our lifetime, but we can take steps to maximize it and to make good use of those new neurons. These new brain cells must be utilized if they are to survive. Neurogenesis alone isn't enough; those new cells must be stimulated and nourished.

Aerobic exercise stimulates neurogenesis—it both creates and nourishes new brain cells. It also increases the level of the hormone BDNF in the brain, which helps those new cells thrive through a process called neuroplasticity, the ability of the brain to form neural connections.

Certain exercises are more effective than others. As you'll see below, not all exercises are created equal. There are certain types of aerobic movement that are much more effective at generating and stimulating new brain cells to build new neuropathways that can create cognitive reserve.

Ready to learn what you can do today to start building brain health? Get ready to jump in—literally!

Move, Eat, and Sleep

Neurogenesis and neuroplasticity are big words, perhaps ones you haven't heard before. That's why what we tell you next is such good news. Contrary to what you might be thinking, you don't have to do anything foreign or unusual to contribute to both.

In fact, the three biggest factors to neurogenesis and neuroplasticity are activities you're already doing in some way, shape, or form. We're talking about how you move, how you eat, and how you sleep. These three behavioral categories are the keys to strengthening brain health and contributing to cognitive (and physical) reserves. We'll discuss each one, in turn, looking at how you can easily enhance your lifestyle and your ability to live the life you deserve, well into the future.

Two Are Better than One

The idea that exercise is good for you is not news. Everyone from Oprah to Dr. Sanjay Gupta to Arnold (Schwarzenegger, of course) is touting the benefits of moving your body. And while any bodily movement is better than none, you need specific types of physical activity if your goal is to increase brain health and contribute to your cognitive reserve.

Specifically, you want to engage in exercise that both generates new brain cells (neurogenesis) AND stimulates those brain cells (neuroplasticity). This is called dual-task exercise.

Our Activate Brain & Body process emphasizes dual-tasking exercises. They are the most efficient forms of exercise because they increase cognitive and physical reserves at the same time. You don't need to buy specialized exercise equipment or learn complicated sports or new hobbies.

In fact, many popular physical activities—some of which you're likely already participating in—are ideal dual-tasking exercises. Here are a few of our favorites.

The Walk of Life

One of the biggest objections to joining a fitness center is that many people feel like they already have to be in shape to go. They think if they can't hit a seven-minute mile on the treadmill or bench press their weight, they better stay home. Unfortunately, that's a huge catch-22. You want to get in shape, so you want to join a gym, but you don't think you're in good enough shape to join a gym. No wonder so many people give up before they get started!

Fortunately, assuming you've gotten the go-ahead from your doctor or medical practitioner, there's absolutely nothing stopping you from getting started right now.

Let's cut to the chase: If you do nothing else, the one thing you absolutely must do is walk.

Walking is, literally and figuratively, the first step to better brain health. From increased circulation to better sleep to lower stress to a longer life, it's hard to overstate the benefits from merely standing up and putting one foot in front of the other.

Walking is the most accessible and simplest exercise you can do. It is, without question, the best exercise for overall health and wellness. It has great aerobic benefits and also builds endurance and leg strength, which helps with core strength and overall balance. It boosts your energy level and immune system and has a minimal chance of leading to injury.

Walking is accessible for most people, even those who don't consider themselves the least bit active. Start by going for a 20-minute brisk walk each day. Add a minute or two each subsequent day, and you can quickly move from being a completely sedentary person to someone who walks a mile, two miles, three miles, or more—just by increasing your distance and pace a bit over time.

One note: To engage your brain, skip the treadmill! While it's better than nothing, when you're walking on a treadmill, every step is predictable. You don't even have to think. You can zone out and listen to music or watch a video. But that's not providing the cognitive challenge we want.

Get outside where you're forced to consider the terrain you're walking on. Your brain is engaged by the scenery and activity around you, and you are paying attention. That's when you're dual tasking.

Picking Up the Pace

Most likely, at some point soon, mere walking will not seem like enough exercise. When that happens, you can dial it up a bit. And you should make every effort to up the intensity because that is where the maximum benefits to brain health and longevity lie.

In fact, if you start to walk more intensely, you'll likely live longer as a result. Researchers at the University of Leicester report that fast walkers could live up to 15 years longer than people who move slowly. Our bodies have evolved to walk, and the more you do and the faster you go, the better off you are.[13]

Go for a Hike.

Hiking is one of the most accessible things you can do on your own to get started, and it may be the perfect "put the brain first" physical activity. Hiking is fantastic because, with every step you take, your brain is constantly involved in calculating the next step. You're increasing your heart rate as well, which, as we will discuss, is one of the keys to building brain health.

With hiking, you are simultaneously building new brain cells and incorporating them as part of your central nervous system. In other words, you are laying down a new pathway for your brain cells to go through, much like the way your heart creates additional pathways for blood to go through because of the repetitive demand vigorous exercise places on the cardiovascular system. We're talking about both neurogenesis and angiogenesis here. More to come on these in upcoming chapters!

Activate Brain & Body co-founder and chairman Martin Pazzani has long been a proponent of the benefits of hiking for longevity and brain health. Years before the new neuroscience supported this belief, and long before Activate Brain & Body, he began referring to hiking as "the fountain of youth" and eventually wrote the 2020 book, *The Secrets of Aging Well: Get Outside*, to encourage more brain healthy, longevity building outdoor exercise.

Skip Away!

Skipping may sound a bit silly, but it's an amazing activity. It requires coordination and balance, and because you're jumping with each step, it's a plyometric exercise. Your muscles are performing an explosive effort, and you're raising your heart rate. And as we know from previous chapters, when your heart rate rises, your body releases more BDNF, a building block for cognitive health.

Now, don't think you've got to look like a crazy person, skipping around the entire block! When you're out walking, just add in an interval of 30 seconds of skipping followed by five minutes of walking. As you get more accustomed to that effort, lengthen the skipping and shorten the walking recovery. You'll feel it quickly!

Brain Dancing

Ready for more? Great, because brain health requires stimulation and challenge. And dancing is another way to get there.

By "dancing," we don't mean merely gyrating to the music—though that can be fun and sweat-inducing. If you want to engage your brain and body, structured partner dancing is the way to go. Ballroom, swing...anything where you must coordinate your moves with a partner in time to the music while your heart rate increases is beneficial.

Because you have to think while moving, you're engaging brain and body and activating both.

A recent study published in *The New England Journal of Medicine* compared dancing to other activities, such as reading and doing crossword puzzles. By far, dancing was the most effective at reducing the risk of dementia.[14]

Percent reduction in the risk of dementia:

- Reading 35%
- Crossword puzzles 4x weekly 47%
- Dancing frequently 76%

Dancing has the ability to reduce stress and depression, increase energy, improve flexibility, strength, balance, and endurance, and boost cardiovascular health. It is also excellent at increasing mental capacity by exercising the brain's cognitive processes because it requires dynamic and rapid-fire decision-making, all of which help to build new neural pathways. So grab a partner and hit it!

Garbage In, Garbage Out

Just as it's no surprise that how you move your body affects your overall health, including brain health, what you put into your body can also impact how your brain functions. Put simply, it's impossible to feed your brain properly if you're not feeding your body properly.

While there are volumes (literally) about proper nutrition, we want to make it simple for you. Limit processed and refined foods, don't overindulge, and stick to a largely Mediterranean eating plan. Not only will this keep your heart healthy, but it will also contribute to your brain health.

According to the Mayo Clinic, a Mediterranean diet is based on the eating habits of countries that border the Mediterranean Sea, such as Italy and Greece.[15] In these areas, there's a reliance on plant-based foods, such as whole grains, vegetables, legumes, fruits, nuts, seeds, herbs, and spices, with olive oil as the main source of added fat.

Protein comes from fish and seafood, from a range of plant-based options like nuts, beans, soya, and quinoa, and from dairy and poultry in moderation. Red meat and sugary treats are included only occasionally.

While this is not a cookbook or nutritional guide, here are some general principles:

- Center meals around vegetables, legumes, and whole grains
- Include fish a minimum of twice a week
- Use olive oil instead of butter in cooking
- Skip dessert, or opt for fresh fruit

And while we're talking about what to consume...don't forget good old H2O! Your cells need water. Do you know that statistic about our bodies being 70 percent water? Guess what—your brain is 70 percent water too, and its cells require water to function. Every part of your body needs water to function properly.

For example, water:

- eliminates waste via urination, perspiration, and bowel movements
- maintains your temperature at normal levels
- lubricates joints.

Not consuming enough water creates dehydration—the condition that occurs when your body does not have adequate water to carry out normal body functions. Even mild dehydration can zap your energy and make you tired. One more: it can also make you feel hungrier and prone to consuming unnecessary calories.

Recall in chapter 3 where we talked about exercise creating BDNF that helps build new brain cells? That process requires proper hydration to work at its best. Medical professionals recommend drinking half your body weight in ounces of water. So, if you weigh 150 pounds, you'd aim for 75 ounces of water per day.

Sleep for Brain Health

Do you know how you feel groggy the morning after a restless night? There's a reason for that! Research shows that slow-wave sleep, also called deep sleep, is a crucial stage in the sleep cycle that enables proper brain function and memory.[16] If you're not sleeping, you're going to have trouble thinking. It's really that simple.

Even beyond the morning-after insomnia struggles, new research around the body's glymphatic system shows this little-studied system plays a huge role in maintaining cognitive health through our lifetimes.[17]

You may be familiar with the body's lymphatic system, a process by which the body rids itself of waste and toxins. Now scientists have found that your brain has a similar process called the glymphatic system, which essentially uses the brain's vascular system as a passageway for clearing waste.

It functions mainly while you are asleep, seems to be shut off while you are awake, and serves to eliminate and drain your brain of neurotoxins. If you're not sleeping, neurotoxins can accumulate.

This accumulation results in a build-up of plaque in the brain, which is thought to contribute to a variety of brain pathologies such as

Alzheimer's, much in the same way your cardiovascular system can be clogged up by a poor diet.

The upshot? Get your sleep. Do whatever you need to in order to clock in your seven to nine hours each night—the amount most adults need.

The Bottom Line

Our goal with this chapter is not to overwhelm you but to show you how easy it is to start supporting your brain health, wherever you are and whatever your current health state is. Don't let the amount of information discourage you. The place to start is here, and the time to start is now. Small changes can make a huge impact.

In fact, according to one study[18], just 35 minutes of continuous walking three times a week, combined with a heart-healthy Mediterranean diet, improved the scores on thinking tests of subjects who were experiencing some functional decline. Remember, it's never too late—or too early—to start working towards brain health!

> These first steps, as important as they are, will give you just a taste of what's possible with a guided program such as Activate, which includes robust metrics and feedback and expert coaches to support your efforts.

At Activate Brain & Body, our programming is filled with functional exercises that incorporate agility and flexibility. They are dual-task activities organized into a science-based process using the latest in technology and aimed at working your brain as much as your heart and your body.

In the next chapters, we'll show you how we've taken the latest discoveries in brain science and built an entire protocol based on tracking our participants' improvement. After all, it's hard to improve what you don't measure!

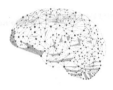

CHAPTER 5

THE TECHNOLOGY OF
BETTER BRAIN HEALTH

*Our philosophy at Activate Brain & Body is for you to compete
only with the previous version of you, not to compete with others
or compare to some unrealistic athletic standard. And so, we
measure everything to keep you on track to reach your goals.*
—MARTIN PAZZANI, CHAIRMAN/
CO-FOUNDER ACTIVATE BRAIN & BODY

Just a decade ago, the idea of wearing a "smartwatch," fitness tracker,
or another personal device that could measure everything from your
calorie expenditure to your heart rate was the stuff of science fiction.

From the invention of the pedometer by Swiss watchmaker Abraham-
Louis Perrelet in 1780 to the introduction of the Fitbit in 2008—yes,
250 years—the technology for wearable fitness devices was relatively
unchanged. But once the Fitbit received widespread attention, the

technology of fitness tracking took off on an exponential growth curve in terms of innovation and adoption.

Now, the worldwide market for "wearable electronics" is expected to hit $265.4 billion by 2026, according to ASD Reports.[19] As a trip to Best Buy or a quick glance at the Apple app store will show, you now have your choice of dozens upon dozens of trackers, apps, gadgets, gizmos, and programs to help you sleep better, eat better, move better, and—their inventors promise—live better.

The devices themselves are evolving so rapidly they now permit medical companies like Doctor on Demand to perform comprehensive medical diagnostics and analysis on patients in remote locations via the internet. Indeed, according to a Facts and Factors market research report, global telemedicine is expected to grow from $40 Billion in 2019 to $475 Billion by 2026[20], stimulating an even bigger boom in DIY self-care diagnostic solutions.

Does Tracking Data Lead to a Better Life?

The ability to track every calorie you eat, every step you take, and every minute you sleep has coalesced into the Quantified Self movement. According to Wikipedia, devotees of this movement share an interest in "self-knowledge through numbers." The thinking is that by using a digital device to track your body, behavior, nutrition, and health, you can improve your mental, physical, and emotional performance. At least that's what the marketers of these devices would like us to believe.

But what is all this data really telling us? Does simply knowing you get an average of 45 minutes of REM sleep per night and walk an average of 6,700 steps each day really mean anything? Will it help you to make concrete, sustainable changes in your behavior that will impact your health in the long run? The answer is maybe ...and maybe not.

A report from Endeavor Partners shows that fitness tracker usage declines over time, from near 100 percent usage on day 1 to less than 50 percent usage at 90 days out.[21] In other words, when you first buy a Fitbit or start using a tracking app, you're all in, often buoyed by the excitement of a new gadget or tech toy. But over time, that excitement and usage wear off.

Experts hypothesize that the drop in usage may be due to the lack of novelty. Once the "fun" wears off, people stop using the technology. Others think that after about 90 days, users have gleaned all the useful information they can from the device, and there's no reason to keep using it because they don't know what to do with the data they've amassed.

Another explanation is that the data is too complicated, and the options are too many. Rather than answering questions, the data generates more uncertainty: Should I track macros or calories? Should I worry about steps or active minutes? Is yoga better for me than tennis?

Turning Technology into Action

If all of this information and the varied options in front of you seem daunting, don't let it deter you. We're your partners in aging well, and we take that role seriously. We at Activate Brain & Body are already diligently researching, testing, applying, and understanding how to optimize the Quantified Self movement.

Our team members live and breathe at the intersection between brain health, body health, and technology, and it's our job to make sense of it for you.

While technology is an incredible tool in the pursuit of brain and body health, it's not the whole picture. If they don't help accomplish the goal of longer, healthier lives, gadgets and devices are simply entertaining distractions. That's why we've distilled the tech into user-friendly tools for you. We want the technology to fade into the background, so the focus is on you and your objectives.

In the next chapter, you'll see how we've combined the best in functional technology with our unique expertise and created what we call The Cognitive Circuit™. This approach allows you to focus on the process while your coach takes care of the tech and the data. The result is a synergistic relationship that will optimize your workouts and your brain and body health.

When this is happening, you are building both cognitive and physical reserves and supporting a happier, healthier, longer life.

Activate Brain & Body is a brain health company, and as is apparent from our name, we put the brain first—always. That's why when you come into one of our centers, you'll immediately notice that the equipment is different from what you'll see at a typical fitness facility.

Everything we offer has been intentionally selected and integrated into The Cognitive Circuit™ to improve brain and body, in that order. If you're looking for intense competition, extreme athletic performance, and/or ultimate activities that cause mental or physical stress, we may not be the right fit for you.

As you'll learn in the next chapters, assessment—and regular reassessments—are critical to charting your path, keeping you motivated, and tracking results.

When you first start, we use the InBody device to provide stats on body composition, including lean body mass. To date, the InBody device has been used in over 2,500 research studies and has proven to be the gold standard in body composition measurement (of course, this information is private and only known to you and your coach).

As you may recall, muscle mass can start to decline in one's 30s, so getting a baseline when you start with Activate plays an important role in how your individual program is customized.

In addition to giving us a baseline for your starting point, the data from this initial assessment is fed into our proprietary algorithm, an equation that calculates an optimal workout plan for you. That algorithm, along with inputs from you and your coach, will determine everything about your customized cognitive circuit program. You'll learn more about the elements of The Cognitive Circuit™ in chapter 6.

After the initial assessment, we'll continue to review and update data approximately every four to eight weeks. That way, we can adjust your plan as needed, account for your progress, and keep you challenged, engaged, and on track to meet your personal goals.

Getting to Know the Tech

Now, let's review some other equipment you might meet during a typical session. By reviewing the state-of-the-art technology, we've chosen to include, you'll soon see how we're different and how you'll get the best of both worlds: high tech AND skilled human coaching.

Myzone

Our measurements don't stop with periodic assessments. Data from each and every one of your workouts is also tracked and recorded in real time. And that's why the Myzone heart rate monitoring system is integral to what goes on inside Activate. Because heart rate is so important to achieving optimal brain and body results, we use this wearable fitness band, which is widely recognized to be a leader in wearable technology and is used by 1.8 million people and over 7500 facilities in 84 countries.

Our philosophy at Activate Brain & Body is that your goal is to strive for your personal best—not to compete with others or reach some unrealistic athletic standard. You will *compete only with the previous version of you*. Myzone supports this goal by tracking effort and comparing your results only with your previous performance.

Cognivue Thrive

The Cognivue Thrive desktop device is a tool for evaluating cognitive function using the same FDA-cleared technology that's been used by neurologists and other physicians. This ten-minute, self-administered computerized screening is simple to implement in our studio by one of our certified brain health trainers.

Cognivue Thrive evaluates three cognitive domains: memory, visuospatial, and executive function. It also measures two important speed performance parameters, reaction time and speed processing. These domains and parameters are key to overall performance at any age and give insight into physical performance as well as your ability to avoid falls and to respond in the correct cognitive manner when undertaking activities such as driving. The results from these five areas make up your personalized Thrive Report, which your coach will use to create your customized workout.

CyberCycle

Cardio is a key component of The Cognitive Circuit™, and while the CyberCycle might resemble a traditional stationary bike, it's so much more. At its core, it is an exercise bike, but it's turbocharged and enhanced with technology to work your brain to provide the dual tasking we've discussed in previous chapters. While you pedal, a large touch screen delivers routines, brain games, and opportunities to challenge your brain while working your body.

The bike is equipped with SmartTouch technology and provides a personalized, interactive cardio workout that challenges both physical and cognitive functioning. Best of all, it's fun. The CyberCycle has even been shown to be superior to traditional exercise in delaying the onset of Alzheimer's and dementia. The *American Journal of Preventive Medicine* supports these findings, writing, "CyberCyclists experienced a 23% reduction in progression to mild cognitive impairment compared to traditional exercisers."[22]

BrainHQ

BrainHQ is the brainchild (no pun intended!) of Posit Science Corporation, an American company providing brain training software and services. The BrainHQ brain-training program is the result of 30 years of research in neurological science and related medicine. Michael Merzenich (a professor emeritus in neurophysiology, member of the National Academy of Sciences, co-inventor of the cochlear implant, and Kavli Prize laureate) led an international team of neuroscientists to design the BrainHQ program.

BrainHQ has more than two dozen online brain exercises that work on attention, brain speed, memory, people skills, navigation, and intelligence. You'll have full access to BrainHQ's range of science-backed cognitive training through a large touch screen at Activate Brain & Body.

The benefits of BrainHQ exercises and assessments have been documented in over 100 published scientific papers. These were independently conducted by scientists at respected universities, including Stanford, the University of California, and Johns Hopkins.[23]

SMARTfit®

Based on the scientific principle of dual-task training, SMARTfit® is the designer and manufacturer of leading professional cognitive-motor training programs. We've talked about this type of training in previous chapters. The unit itself is a large, upright, computerized panel that you'll interact with as part of The Cognitive Circuit™, guided by our coaches.

SMARTfit interactive brain health training offers a unique approach to improving the cognitive and physical health of individuals who usually don't work out or play sports. SMARTfit adds to the power of dual-task training by delivering all activities using gamification, creating an immersive exercise game environment.

The games are easy to learn yet engaging, with enough challenge to trigger the desire to achieve and improve. This game exercise format adds to both engagement and enjoyment.

More Than the Sum of the Parts

Individually, these pieces of equipment are marvels of the latest and greatest creations in the field of brain health technology. But woven together, they're so much more.

They can be used in an infinite variety of arrangements for The Cognitive Circuit™, a system that has one purpose: to activate your brain, energize your body, and ignite your spirit. But this doesn't happen on its own. The pieces must be intentionally and skillfully assembled by an expert in the field of brain and body health. And that's what Activate offers and what your coach imparts to you.

Your coach will work with you personally to create a routine and program to meet your goals by maximizing the production of BDNF each and every time you come into the Activate Brain & Body center. Read on to chapter 6 to see the power of The Cognitive Circuit™ and its ability to improve your life, inside and out.

Then, in chapter 7, we'll share more about what makes the Activate Brain & Body coaches an indispensable part of your overall wellness and health plan.

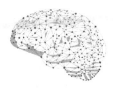

THE COGNITIVE CIRCUIT™: THE CORE OF YOUR SUCCESS

The point of exercise is to build and condition the brain.
—MARIE STONER, CHIEF SCIENCE OFFICER,
CO-FOUNDER, ACTIVATE BRAIN & BODY

Now that you know more about the technology behind Activate Brain & Body, you might be wondering what it's like to actually go through a fully customized brain and body training session.

How is it different from your regular big-box fitness center or your local personal training studio? Will you be hooked up via electrodes to a bank of computer monitors, like something out of a science fiction movie? Not exactly, though the experience might seem a little futuristic at first!

One of the most critical components is the initial assessment. The Activate Brain & Body team members are big believers in collecting and using biometric data. It has been said by many that "You can't manage what you don't measure." We like to take this a step further by saying, "You can't improve what you don't measure."

At your first visit, every new Activate Brain & Body member undergoes a comprehensive screening to create a snapshot of your initial cognitive and physical benchmark. Measurements include everything from body composition, flexibility, and balance, to memory, visuospatial skills, executive function, processing speed, and reaction time. You'll also be asked about your personal goals—be they increased functional strength, body composition, stress relief, cognitive improvements, or all of the above.

Based on this information, your coach will prepare a customized 8-week plan specifically for you. Each time you attend one of your group sessions, your personalized plan is already laid out and ready to go.

When you show up, nothing is random. For the next 60 minutes, you're led through very specific activities, including cardiovascular exercises, resistance activities, and brain training, using some of the technologies like the SMARTfit board we introduced you to in the previous chapter.

You're never left on your own, you never have to guess what to do next, and you're never bored because every session is unique, upbeat, motivating, and fun.

Congratulations! At the end of the hour, you'll have raised your heart rate, burned calories, worked your muscles, challenged your brain and body, and built new brain cells …all while having fun in a supportive group setting. You've just completed your first cognitive circuit, the core of Activate Brain & Body.

What is The Cognitive Circuit™?

The Cognitive Circuit™ is a guided 60-minute workout that will activate your brain, invigorate your body, and ignite your spirit. It is the cornerstone of the Activate Brain & Body program.

We developed it through a decade of trials and test programs, in conjunction with the latest research and input from experts in the fields of aging, neuroscience, fitness, nutrition, and stress management. **The result: a unique, brain-first approach to building cognitive and physical reserves to allow you to take control of the way you age.**

The concept behind The Cognitive Circuit™ is based on what we now know to be true about brain health. By undertaking specific activities in a specific sequence, you can prime your brain for neurogenesis (creation of new brain cells) and neuroplasticity (networking and connections of brain cells).

The Cognitive Circuit™ is comprised of three components:
- **Metabolic stations** to raise the heart rate, burn calories, and activate the brain-derived neurotrophic factor (BDNF) we spoke about in previous chapters.

- **Dual tasking**, using cognitively loaded resistance training to challenge the body and the brain simultaneously.

- **Focused brain training** to engage your brain with a variety of problem-solving games and dual tasking while the heart rate is elevated.

Let's look at each of these and its role in The Cognitive Circuit™.

Metabolic Station

As you now know from previous chapters, aerobic exercise is a critical component of brain health. Research shows that achieving a heart rate of 65–75 percent of maximum is ideal for release of BDNF, the brain's protein that promotes the survival of nerve cells (neurons). In fact, under these conditions, BDNF levels can increase two- to three-fold!

You will achieve the ideal heart rate range through a combination of functional exercises that replicate real-life situations, so what you do in your workout will have a direct correlation to the activities in your daily life.

Cognitively Loaded Resistance Training

Research shows that aerobic activity is wonderful for cardiovascular health and for burning calories. And while it can lead to higher levels of BDNF, it's not a good workout for your brain on its own. That's where resistance training comes in. Using kettlebells, exercise bands, and your own bodyweight, you'll challenge your muscles in new and different ways.

You might be asked to combine a single leg with a single arm, moving in different planes of motion—moving forward, backward, and sideways in different combinations to keep your mind and body guessing.

In this module, you'll also be cognitively challenged through movement as well as brain tasks. The goal is dual tasking: to introduce a new challenge to both brain and body, so the new brain cells created in the metabolic station are incorporated into new neural pathways, adding to your cognitive reserve.

By having your heart rate elevated while participating in a novel activity, perhaps at the SMARTfit board, the new brain cells being formed are more likely to remain and connect to the various domains (memory, visuospatial, etc.) to help build cognitive reserve.

Brain Training

The third component of The Cognitive Circuit™ is brain training, which is the focus of every workout. This is accomplished through new skill acquisition using foreign movements most people aren't familiar with. By mixing up activities and continuing to challenge your brain in new and different ways, you'll be building new brain cells and immediately incorporating them into new neural networks.

At the end of your session, you can leave knowing you've given yourself a top-to-bottom workout designed to help you continue to live a long and healthy life …on your terms.

Beyond the Core

The Cognitive Circuit™ may be at the core of our work at Activate Brain & Body, but there's more. Every element of your experience with us will have been carefully and intentionally designed to support brain health and the development of cognitive and physical reserves.

Your workout starts with the brain. All of our programming is centered around the brain, and for good reason. From the structure of our sessions to the design of our studio, all decisions and exercises are based on a "brain first" model. By prioritizing the brain first (the opposite of the vast majority of current approaches to whole-body fitness), we ensure that your brain is primed to take advantage of the neurogenesis brought about by physical effort.

Yes, our workouts all have a physical component (and you will see increases in your physical performance), but it's all in service of creating cognitive reserve. We're not a fitness studio; we're a brain health center.

Your Program Is Customized to YOU

Examine any two brain scans, even those of identical twins, and you'll see significant differences. Your brain isn't like anyone else's, and neither is your body. That's why we create a customized program based on your current assessment and your personal goals. While you're participating in a group session, everything is tailored to you—where you are and where you want to be.

Many of the activities we use within The Cognitive Circuit™ are the same as those used by high-level athletes to increase their response time, decision-making abilities, and recovery. But you don't need to be a professional athlete to benefit from these techniques. These same activities are also used with individuals experiencing cognitive issues, such as those recovering from traumatic brain injuries (TBIs), concussions, and dementia.

Our program can make your life better, whatever your starting point. We meet you where you are.

1. **Your progress is consistently measured and tracked.**
    Tracking is critical, not only for assessment but for motivation as well. When we look at brain function, progress is not linear and is not always noticeable in a real-life setting. That's why an initial assessment and regular follow-up assessments at 8-week intervals are critical. These allow you to easily track your progress, even if it's not immediately apparent in your everyday life. This helps keep you motivated and committed to the process...because you'll see the results!

2. **Your experience is enhanced with a group setting.**
    While it's possible to undertake many of these activities on your own, research has shown that working out in a group has many added benefits. From friendly competition to mutual

support and encouragement, participating in group exercise is simply more enjoyable—which means you're more likely to stick with it.

In one study, people who exercised in a group rather than on their own had decreased stress levels and had better mental and physical well-being at the end of a 12-week fitness program.[24]

Additionally, socialization is one of the key components of healthy aging. Study after study confirms what we know intuitively: Relationships are critical to our health, including our brain health. In a study at the Mesulam Center for Cognitive Neurology and Alzheimer's Disease at Northwestern University Feinberg School of Medicine, scientists found that "SuperAgers," defined as people aged 80 and above who had the mental agility of much younger people, appeared to have one thing in common—close friends.[25]

At Activate Brain & Body, our members are encouraged to connect through a number of opportunities, from wine tastings and cooking classes to seminars and group check-ins.

3. **Your program incorporates stress reduction.**
    It's hard to open a health magazine or browse a fitness website without seeing a reference to "inflammation."[26] It seems to be the latest buzzword, with good reason. Inflammation is your body's attempt to protect you from infection. But when your body's protective instincts go into overdrive, it can lead to chronic inflammation, which, in turn, is related to cancer, heart disease, diabetes, and Alzheimer's disease.

    And one of the key contributors to chronic inflammation is stress. Chronic stress releases cortisol, which has been shown to raise blood glucose levels. Additionally, stress hormones can damage neurons, especially their connections. And prolonged exposure to extreme stress can lead to major atrophy of the hippocampus and neuronal death—the exact opposite of what we want to do via neurogenesis!

At Activate Brain & Body, we want to help you address anything that can be offsetting your brain health—and that includes stress. As part of your Activate Brain & Body membership, you'll receive access to stress management sessions and tools, where we use a combination of equipment, breathing exercises, and physical approaches to relieve tension in your body and decrease overall cortisol levels.

The Secret Sauce

Does this all sound like a lot? It is. But don't let that put you off. One of the key differentiators when you come to Activate Brain & Body is the fact that you get to just "show up."

You don't need to become an expert at neurogenesis or cortisol reduction. You don't have to track your own progress. You don't have to keep up with the latest research in nutrition, neuroscience, and exercise physiology. That's our job.

And that brings us to one of the most critical elements of Activate Brain & Body—our coaches. Our staff of carefully selected and thoroughly skilled certified brain health trainers is our secret sauce, serving as your point of contact, instructor, encourager, and guide. These coaches are so important, we've devoted an entire chapter to their specialized role.

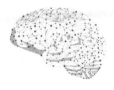

CHAPTER 7

YOUR COACH TIES IT ALL TOGETHER

In the future, your fitness coach will be as
important as your financial planner.
—SPECIAL REPORT, *THE WALL STREET JOURNAL*

Actually, at Activate Brain & Body, we believe your fitness coach may be *more* important than your financial planner.

If you own a business, you probably have an expert financial planner or accountant who knows how to optimize current financial laws and regulations and who prepares your quarterly reporting and annual taxes.

If you have ever been involved in a real estate transaction, you probably worked with a real estate agent who handles the paperwork and details of the purchase or sale to make sure things proceed quickly and legally. If you want to build a house, you'll deal with an architect, an engineer, and a general contractor—not to mention the plumbers, electricians, painters, landscapers, and possibly an interior designer or two.

There are specialists who match students with the right colleges. There are specialists for selecting the right color for your home's exterior. There are specialists in everything from applying for a government small business grant to writing a can't-miss profile for your favorite dating app. We've become a nation of specialists!

It's understandable. As the amount of information available to us has skyrocketed, so has our overwhelm. The simple truth is, we can't be authorities on everything. And most of us simply don't have the time to stay on top of the latest discoveries in all the fields we're interested in.

That's why it's critical to find trusted experts who can guide us, motivate us, provide feedback, keep us accountable, and keep on top of emerging research and best practices in fields we care about.

And that's exactly what our Activate Brain & Body coaches do for our members. In every human endeavor, the best results occur when you have a coach.

What Exactly IS a Coach?

The term "coach" is thrown around indiscriminately these days. From corporate coaches to life coaches to professional sports coaches, there is no one definition.

But at Activate Brain & Body, when we refer to our coaches, we use the term very intentionally and very specifically. Our team members hold a number of nationally accredited fitness and nutrition certifications, including:

- Functional Aging Specialist (FAS)
- National Academy of Sports Medicine (NASM)
- Corrective Exercise Specialist (NASM CES)
- Precision Nutrition Certification (PN)
- Brain Health Trainer (BHT)

At Activate Brain & Body, our coaches are indispensable. From your first visit, you'll experience the difference in terms of their knowledge, their ability to translate complex scientific concepts into easy-to-understand instructions, and their dedication to helping you achieve your individual goals. And it all starts with the assessment.

> Our Coaches: Highly experienced, qualified, and trained individuals who understand the brain and the body and are committed to supporting our members in their quest to achieve the highest levels of brain health.

Your Assessment

We talked a bit in the last chapter about how each member is assessed at the beginning of their program and then monitored constantly along the way. This initial assessment is where it all begins because tracking and monitoring progress is key to our entire program.

In addition to recording your baseline cognitive and physical metrics, your coach also will discuss your personal goals and objectives. Do you want enough stamina for that trip to Disney with your kids or grandkids? Do you want to keep working into your 70s and 80s? What do you envision your later years to look like, and are you on the path to get there? And if not, what adjustments need to be made now to ensure you're on track to meet or exceed your goals?

Once your assessment is complete, your coach will use the data we've collected, the results of our proprietary algorithm, and his/her expertise to map out a specific plan for you over your next eight weeks. **It's a well-thought-out process, unlike anything else—the best of both worlds, where the latest high-tech tools meet human expertise.**

Your plan is customized to you and your movement pattern, not how "in shape" you are. Much like when a doctor prescribes medicine, your coach will recommend exercises and a program based on specific data gathered from your assessment. But you don't have to worry about the details (unless you're interested in the nitty-gritty—and some people are!). You just need to show up and get to work.

Accountability and Motivation

Speaking of showing up…there's a false belief that knowledge is enough to move intelligent people to action. Unfortunately, that's not true. Humans are experts at avoiding discomfort, holding tight to what's familiar, and justifying a lack of forward momentum.

And that's the power of a coach: they step into the gap between knowing and doing. By taking an interest in you and holding you accountable to your goals, your coach vastly increases your likelihood of sticking with your program. In fact, statistics show that people who work with a fitness coach get better results, with fewer injuries, and are more likely to make lifestyle changes that last.[27]

There's been a lot of buzz lately about the use of technology in fitness (which you saw in chapter 5). As exciting and groundbreaking as these innovations are, the myriad of technological tools has distracted from a few fundamental truths about human behavior.

People tend to get bored quickly with new equipment and technology, and typically, after just a few months, their interest starts to wane.

What at the start was a two-to-three-times-a-week habit drops to once or twice a week, and then to once or twice a month.

Without even realizing it, you've lost your motivation, and the subsequent lack of results further drains your willingness to get back to the routine. You've dropped off …and at a regular fitness center, that might be the end of it. But not at Activate Brain & Body.

Leading-edge technology will always be a part of Activate Brain & Body and The Cognitive Circuit™. However, the human element of working with a high-quality coach is something that technology still doesn't have an answer for. That's why we rely on our uniquely skilled and trained coaches to create the best of both worlds—high tech and high touch.

On those days when you just don't feel like showing up, your coach is there to encourage you, show you how far you've come, and remind you of why you got started. They're also willing to have the hard conversations when appropriate, in service of your mental and physical health.

Support and Guidance

One of the most important functions of a coach is to ensure you're performing exercises and activities correctly, thereby minimizing the possibility of injury and maximizing results. Particularly when working with unfamiliar technology or equipment, we want to make sure you know what you're doing and how to do it safely. That means also understanding why we've included certain activities in The Cognitive Circuit™.

But as we've said, it doesn't mean you have to be an expert. Much of the information you're learning about the brain can be new and initially hard to grasp. That's what your coach is here for. Your coach is your guide on your Activate Brain & Body journey. They run interference between the science and your sessions in the center. When you're confused, they're on hand to explain—with empathy, not criticism.

Our team realizes that brain and body fitness are based on incremental progress, taken one step at a time. And it's not always going to be easy. Your coach is there to meet you where you are, addressing any issues that may be getting in the way of your goals, whether they occur inside or outside the facility.

Care, Not Competition

At Activate Brain & Body, our emphasis is on working as a team with our clients. We're all working together with a common goal. Many of our team members have friends or family members who have experienced cognitive or physical decline before their time, and they are now committed to helping others achieve optimal brain and body health so they can avoid that fate.

Our coaches know that it's not about being the best in the workout or finishing the workout the fastest. Our goal is to work together with our members towards a healthier, more enjoyable life. When you join us, you can be assured you're never alone in the pursuit of your goals.

In sum, forget everything you know about coaches in the fitness industry. Activate Brain & Body coaches are a different breed, consistently striving to learn more, grow more, and make a larger impact within the community.

They use the latest technology and work with a process that ensures you will get the best of both worlds: the latest curated brain health technology and the leading edge of human coaching and motivation.

And, they never forget that they have an incredible opportunity to show up and make a life-changing difference—for you.

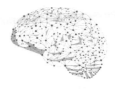

CHAPTER 8

WHEN YOU PUT YOUR BRAIN FIRST, YOUR BODY FOLLOWS

You know you've got to exercise your brain just like your muscles.
—WILL ROGERS

As we've repeated numerous times to this point, we put the brain first. Everything we've developed—our programs featuring The Cognitive Circuit™, our extensive coach training, even the interior design of our facility—is designed to create and optimize brain health. But that does not mean we neglect the body—quite the contrary.

To our amazement and delight, over the course of our years of trial programs and research, we discovered that when you put the brain first, not only does the body follow, but the body thrives in ways that are exactly what aging bodies need.

Not only that, but by following our brain and body fitness programs, you're not going to get bulked up like a bodybuilder. What's going to happen is that every important measure of physiological and functional fitness that matters to you is going to improve. We'll talk a lot about that in this chapter.

No matter what level of fitness you are now, Activate Brain & Body has a program for you. And it's never too late (or too soon) to start.

If things are pretty good for you already, being "activated" makes it all better. You'll most likely have more spring in your step, walk a little faster, and have a more positive outlook. You'll probably feel sharper, more focused, and more alert. Your sleep may improve, your resting heart rate may go down, and your endurance and flexibility will most definitely benefit.

If things aren't going so well right now, being "activated" can give you the willpower, the energy, and the confidence to turn it around. Being fit allows you to access your full potential—to unleash the best version of yourself and to experience and participate more fully in every aspect of your life.

Being fit the Activate Brain & Body way is not just about recreational activities and playing sports. Being 'activated' permits you to function more effectively in the world: lift a suitcase into the overhead bin, shovel snow, rearrange the furniture, carry a box of books up the stairs, walk the dog, go surfing and skiing, play tennis or pickleball, drive your car more alertly, and so on.

All of these activities are helped by functional fitness training, which is one of the cornerstones of our program. Functional fitness strengthens and trains your muscles to work together, preparing them not only for the things you do every day but for the activities you've planned in the years ahead.

And being activated keeps you independent and, of course, active. If you want to work into your 70s or take on a new career, you can. If you want to travel the world, you can do it more easily. If you want to walk across Spain on the Camino de Santiago Trail or hike sections of the Appalachian Trail, you'll be able to. How about this: if you want to go for a long daily walk in the park with your great-grandchildren, you can do that as well.

Another invaluable benefit likely to result from attaining a new, higher level of fitness: you will likely avoid exhausting your life savings and retirement benefits on medical expenses, and you won't spend the last ten years of your life drugged up, being driven from one doctor's office to another. Being fit and active now gives you the best chance for a different and better outcome for your later years.

Taking charge of the way you age really comes down to the choices you make. Numerous studies have documented the brain and body benefits that can happen if you embrace the idea of making lifestyle choices that can have profound effects on your health.

The Benefits Can Be Enormous

The following sections detail just some of the brain and body benefits you can look forward to if you embrace the idea of taking charge of the way you age. By committing to improving your fitness now, you will add to your physical and cognitive reserves, and you will likely enjoy a longer—and perhaps more important—healthier life.

Fit People Have Bigger Brains

After the age of 40, the average human brain naturally begins to shrink, typically by about five percent per year. However, people who maintain a high degree of fitness are able to drastically slow and reverse the deterioration. Being fit has great benefits for your brain.[28]

Conversely, an obese person's brain can be up to eight percent smaller than a fit person's. Research at the Cleveland Clinic looked at people with an average age of 55 and found that a high percentage of body fat is linked to having a smaller brain.[29] Being sedentary and obese can literally shrink your brain.

Fit People Are Healthier in General

The more frequently you exercise and the more intense that exercise is, the greater the health benefits. Intense exercise also significantly reduces the likelihood of cancer, diabetes, dementia, stroke, and cardiovascular disease. Fit people who do weight-bearing exercise build stronger bones, making them more resistant to falls and other accidents.[30]

Being Fit Can Give Your Immune System a Boost

Consistent exercise results in a stronger immune system—a bonus that is supported by numerous studies. One investigation found that even moderate exercise appears to have a "beneficial effect on the immune function, which could protect against upper respiratory tract infections."[31]

The benefits are especially helpful as you get older since your immune system declines as you age. The more you exercise, the more blood and oxygen course through your body, and that creates a powerful anti-inflammatory effect. It makes your body stronger and better able to fight off a variety of illnesses.

Reduced Flu and Pneumonia Deaths

Viral respiratory infections represent the most common form of infectious disease and account for over seven percent of all deaths.[32] Deaths associated with respiratory viral infections occur most often in the elderly and other immune-compromised individuals whose immune systems are incapable of handling an elevated viral load. Researchers have found that "prolonged, intense exercise causes immunosuppression, while moderate-intensity exercise improves immune function and potentially reduces risk and severity of respiratory viral infection."[33]

Based on available evidence, moderate-intensity exercise training should be used as an adjunct to other preventative measures against respiratory tract viral infection.[34] In a world where we're now all acutely aware of respiratory viruses, we find this to be an important study.

Fit People Live Longer

There is now science-based evidence that as little as 15 minutes of exercise each day can have tremendous longevity benefits. There is also clear statistical evidence that not exercising at all significantly increases your risk of an early death. More compelling is the research being done on the older population. The Human Performance Laboratory at Ball State University discovered that "people in their 70s who exercise regularly can have the heart, lung, and muscle fitness of healthy people 30 years younger."[35]

Another report in the *British Journal of Sports Medicine* indicates that exercise can be spaced out throughout a full day and that even 10 minutes of vigorous exercise, here and there, have a clear impact on life span.[36] Just think about that for a second and realize how easy it would be to add two or three 10-minute bursts of physical activity to your day.

It's Never Too Late to Start

Studies now show unfit people as old as age 79 who have never exercised can receive significant benefits by increasing their activity level and beginning an exercise program. Inactive people at that age decreased their mortality rate by 24 percent with an increase in physical activity. "There are clearly benefits at all levels" of activity, said lead researcher Dr. Soren Brage, a principal investigator with the MRC Epidemiology Unit at the University of Cambridge. "The most encouraging thing is you don't have to be a super-athlete, and it's never too late."[37]

Decreased Chance of Heart Disease

The fitter you are, the less likely you are to suffer from any kind of heart disease. Increasing your fitness level strengthens the heart muscle and significantly reduces the chance of cardiovascular illnesses, like heart attacks, clogged arteries (atherosclerosis), or hardening of the arteries (arteriosclerosis). A strong heart muscle also improves circulation to your entire body, which benefits all of your bodily organs and processes.

Reduced Likelihood of Hypertension

High blood pressure is part of the metabolic syndrome cluster of symptoms. Untreated high blood pressure can lead to stroke, heart attack, kidney disease, and early dementia. It is most often treated with a program of long-term medication. In many of these cases (specifically the ones not associated with a genetic component), regular physical activity can prevent, reduce, and control blood pressure.

Diminished Diabetes

Diabetes is a disease in which your body's ability to produce or respond to insulin is weakened. Insulin is a hormone that regulates blood glucose (sugar), which is a source of energy for the body. There are two forms of diabetes—type 1 and type 2. Both result in elevated levels of glucose in the blood and urine, and they have several symptoms in common, including frequent urination, increased thirst and hunger, fatigue, and numbness in hands and feet.

Type 1 diabetes is an autoimmune disorder where the body attacks and destroys the cells that produce insulin. Type 2 diabetes is a metabolic syndrome disorder—either the body doesn't produce enough insulin, or the insulin that is produced doesn't work the way it should.

Obesity is a significant risk factor for developing type 2 diabetes. Studies have shown that an obese person is up to 80 times more likely to develop type 2 diabetes than those with a leaner body type.[38] Further, structured exercise has been shown to improve glycemic control, i.e., it can improve the body's ability to manage energy resources.[39]

Decreased Risk of Cancer

In a landmark 2016 study, American Cancer Society and National Cancer Institute researchers found that exercise was associated with a significantly decreased risk of colon cancer, breast cancer, endometrial cancer, esophageal cancer, liver cancer, stomach cancer, kidney cancer, and myeloid leukemia. The study found that this was due, in part, to the fact that exercise helps with weight management; however, exercise was also found to help better regulate hormones, insulin levels, and the immune system. Physical activity was found to be "strongly associated with a decreased risk of multiple myeloma, a blood cancer, as well as cancers of the head and neck, rectum, bladder, and lung (in current and former smokers)."[40]

The Mayo Clinic in Rochester, Minnesota, even goes so far as to call exercise a secret weapon and one of the most important elements of cancer treatment. Sara Mansfield, M.S., a certified cancer exercise trainer with the Mayo Clinic Healthy Living Program, says, "Physical activity can help people before, during, and after cancer treatment. Research tells us, in general, it's better to move more than less."[41]

Fighting Sarcopenia

This condition results from a gradual loss of muscle, including muscle mass, strength, size, quality/elasticity, power, and stamina. It typically begins during your forties. Simply put, it is the weakness we associate with aging and largely the result of age plus inactivity. It happens so gradually that it's hard to notice until, all of a sudden, you're frail. Your muscles have shriveled, and your bones are unprotected and brittle.

The good news is that the onset of sarcopenia can be delayed for many years, and it is a somewhat reversible condition. Resistance training and weight-bearing exercises are essential to prevent and slow the advance of sarcopenia. With proper exercise, it is even possible to reverse it. According to Nathan LeBrasseur of Mayo Clinic, "Without question, exercise is the most powerful intervention to address muscle loss, whether it occurs in the context of advancing age or debilitating chronic or acute diseases."[42]

More Body Benefits

As we've stated, when you put the brain first, the body thrives in ways that are exactly what aging bodies need.

But wait, there's more!

Throughout the course of our research and trial programs, we've extensively interviewed participants, both before they began training and after a few months of participating in our cognitive workout programs. They report:

- Improved sense of balance and coordination

- Increased flexibility and range of motion

- Increased endurance, stamina, and energy

- Improved quality and duration of sleep

- Feeling less overwhelmed and more able to take on the day

- Reduced feelings of stress/anxiety and improved mood

- Feeling refreshed, rejuvenated, and invigorated

All this adds up to one of our key goals: enabling people to live longer, happier, healthier lives. And it all starts with putting your brain first.

What happens to your body when you put the brain first?

It's like getting your superpowers back.

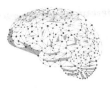

CHAPTER 9

REINVENTING FITNESS AS UPSTREAM PREVENTIVE HEALTHCARE

The fitness industry is one of the most profitable and persuasive businesses out there, but in terms of promised results, it has been a disappointing failure. There are very few fitness brands, technologies and commercial programs which actually deliver what they promise.
—SINDHUJAA KUMAR IN *ENTREPRENEUR MAGAZINE*, 2018

Throughout the book, we have been using the phrase "you can take charge of the way you age." That's because science clearly shows that certain types of physical and cognitive exercises build brain health and that when you put your brain first, your body follows.

The implications of this, when you think about it, are vast and profound: How long will I live? What will be the quality of the years in the last one-third of my life? Will I outlive my resources? Will I need family and friends to support me? What will I be capable of doing in my 70s, 80s, and 90s?

Prevention is the Key

Avoiding, delaying, or minimizing physical and cognitive decline is the impetus that compelled us to create Activate Brain & Body and what drives us to share what we know about creating better brain and body health in the pursuit of happier, healthier, and longer lives. We believe we can make a difference.

The only true preventive healthcare—where prevention is defined as "the action of stopping something from happening"—occurs long before you show symptoms. It happens long before you need the medical/pharma system and long before you go to the doctor with a problem. This prevention is the result of the way you live your life, the choices you make, how and what you eat, and, especially, how you approach fitness.

The traditional way of defining prevention divides the concept into three parts:

1. **Tertiary Prevention**, which attempts to reduce the damage done by a symptomatic disease. This focuses on rehabilitation and managing disabilities, reducing the symptoms without dealing with the underlying cause of the disease. This includes things like medicines prescribed for COPD, heart conditions, and to ease the pain of terminal cancers.

2. **Secondary Prevention**, which attempts to prevent an asymptomatic disease from progressing to a symptomatic disease. This area receives a lot of attention, and it is now often described as "a pill for everything."

3. Primary Prevention, which means life and behavioral choices that prevent disease and are nonclinical. This is what we mean by upstream preventive healthcare, and it's where nutrition and fitness belong. This is where we believe the long-term solutions lie: reducing and preventing the need for massive resources spent on Tertiary and Secondary prevention.

Primary prevention is where we operate, an area that we—and other forward-thinking innovators—are calling upstream preventive healthcare. We've made it our mission to reinvent, redefine, and elevate fitness with that in mind. Does that mean we classify ourselves as a healthcare company? No, primary prevention means lifestyle and behavior choices that are scientifically shown to reduce the probability of disease. By no means are an Activate Brain & Body membership and programs intended to substitute for medical advice, diagnosis, or treatment.

A Curious and Disappointing Correlation

The fitness industry boom of the last generation is not making us fitter as a population. The advent of large, corporate fitness companies, while useful places to get fit for some, also coincides with a massive obesity epidemic, as well as exponential increases in diabetes and other symptoms of metabolic syndrome such as high blood pressure.

So, something is out of whack. To some, fitness might even be considered a failed business model—overdue for upgrades required to provide service to a broader population. But there is hope for the fitness business if we can evolve the industry because it has so much to offer in the area of primary prevention.

The problem, from our perspective, is that much of the industry is myopically focused on the young demographic, and it does not focus nearly enough on outcomes that are more than simply how you look. It's been too concerned with merely acquiring new members and opening more and more facilities. In this case, quantity does not equal quality.

Let's look at the facts.

In 1960, roughly the start of the organized fitness business, when there were fewer than 3000 fitness clubs across America, the percentage of the population that were fitness club members was very small. Now, more than 60 years later, there are 50,000 fitness centers with 64 million paying members. The data clearly shows that overall, as a nation, we are much less fit and much less active than we were in 1960.[43]

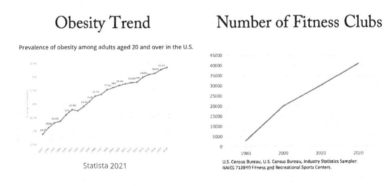

Figure 4. The growth in obesity mirrors the growth in the number of fitness clubs. Correlation like this does not mean causation, but it does show the industry's ineffectiveness at a population level.

Healthcare costs are rising, with no sign of slowing down anytime soon:

- National health expenditures grew by 5% to $3.8 trillion in 2019. That amounts to $11,582 spent per person and accounts for 17.7% of the gross domestic product (GDP).

- Out of pocket spending grew 4.6% to $406.5 billion in 2019 or 11% of total healthcare expenditure.

- Prescription drug spending increased 5.7% to $369.7 billion in 2019, up from a 3.8% growth in 2018.[44]

The costs to care for an unfit and rapidly aging population are massive and have grown to become a dominant factor in the U.S. economy. It is important to note that all of these statistics are pre-pandemic—the impact of which has yet to be fully calculated:

- National health spending is projected to grow at an average annual rate of 5.4% for 2019-28 and reach $6.2 trillion by 2028.

- Price growth for medical goods and services is projected to accelerate, averaging 2.4% per year for 2019–28 (partly reflecting an expected faster growth in health sector wages).

- Per-person, personal healthcare spending for the 65 and older population was $19,098 in 2014, over five times higher than spending per child ($3,749) and almost three times the spending per working-age person ($7,153).

- Those considered elderly were the smallest population group, nearly 15% of the population, yet they accounted for approximately 34 % of all spending in 2014.[45]

What this adds up to is an unaffordable scenario that will bankrupt people, companies, and countries. **According to AARP, older Americans are prescribed, on average, four and one-half prescriptions per month.** If brand-name drugs (not generics) are used to treat chronic conditions, the average annual retail cost for that number of medications in 2017 would be approximately $30,591 per person.[46]

We know there's a better way. We have to take control of our personal health, and that means looking beyond prescriptions. Of course, if a medication is needed, it should be taken. But maintaining physical health—upstream prevention—must become a more important part of the equation. Doctors should be able to write prescriptions for fitness memberships, walking, hiking, biking, and more. It would make all of us healthier.

A Pill for Everything?

We have amazing new medical and pharmacological innovations, unimaginable only a generation ago, that can extend life and stall once-fatal diseases. But at the same time, we are all concerned about the increasingly high cost, availability, and limitations of healthcare. And we're also increasingly skeptical of a medical and pharmacological business model that often views us not as patients but as long-term, living, recurring revenue streams. Someone on blood pressure or anti-cholesterol meds at age 40 could remain on medications for the next 30-plus years.

Sadly, the fitness industry is still struggling, despite its size and ubiquity, to play a respected role in making the culture healthier and fitter. We have seen this ourselves as insiders.

To some, the fitness industry is seen as one of high-pressure sales, deceptive and unclear membership agreements, uncomfortable or intimidating membership experiences, predatory or untrained club employees, unclean/germy places, and more.

So while our roots are in fitness, we are also critics of it, and we are determined to elevate fitness to become the key linchpin in creating a fitter, healthier world. The fitness industry should aspire to be the solution to the simmering, never-ending, and seemingly unsolvable healthcare crisis that the aging population is only accelerating.

What we are talking about by focusing on upstream prevention is macro-level change—the kind of change that can take the pressure off of the healthcare system, reduce healthcare expenses associated with poor lifestyle choices, and decrease the reliance on health insurance providers to come to the rescue.

The Activate model is different from traditional fitness businesses and aspires to do just that. Our model requires:

- A rigorous, science-based approach that also understands human motivation and behavior

- The measurement and assessment of key brain and body metrics

- A focus on programs and behaviors that get results

- An understanding of how to gain compliance and coach people toward a longer health span

It's about re-engineering the experiential, motivational, and social aspects of a business that has not delivered on its promise nor served the needs of an aging population.

We believe your fitness goals should include the bonus of providing you with actual upstream preventive healthcare. It occurs so far upstream that you cannot see or hear the waterfalls or rapids. It happens before you have the early signs of cognitive decline, before you have symptoms like shortness of breath or hypertension, or before you have an expanded waistline.

We believe it's time to begin the transition to thinking ahead and starting early. Doctors need to add prescriptions for fitness to their treatment plans, and healthcare insurance companies need to support this effort.

By focusing on upstream prevention, not only might we prevent, delay, or minimize common aging maladies from occurring, but we also save healthcare expenses and make your life better.

There is no magic pill.

Who makes money on upstream prevention? Well, you do, actually.

If you prevent yourself from getting sick, becoming obese, developing any aspect of metabolic syndrome, or sliding into cognitive decline, you will spend less on medical care over the course of your lifetime. So, you have more money. Simple. The best way to get this far upstream is fitness. And the best way to get the maximum benefit of this fitness is to start now to take charge of the way you age.

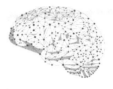

CHAPTER 10

UPSTREAM PREVENTION IN PRACTICE

Prevention is better than cure.
—DESIDERIUS ERASMUS

What we like best about focusing on real upstream prevention, beyond the fact that it saves people from expensive medical issues: *it is really about each individual being empowered with the knowledge and resources to live their best life.*

Although not enough focus is placed on prevention at present, it is far from a new concept. Benjamin Franklin famously said in 1736, "an ounce of prevention is worth a pound of cure." Although at the time, he was speaking of fire prevention measures, he understood that taking precautions in the present was far preferable to suffering severe consequences much later on.

Unfortunately, the human psyche seems to always be in denial that something bad can happen to us until it happens, and then we try to reverse and undo it. For some reason, and against all logic, most people make a few bad lifestyle choices (some make a lot of them) that contribute directly to their own significant and expensive illnesses, disease, and death.

According to *Psychology Today*, "The problem with reinforcing preventive behaviors is that the reward not only comes too long after the desired behavior (years or even decades) but that it comes in the form of something that *fails to happen*."[47]

Only when a health problem surfaces and there are symptoms to react to do we try to fix it. By then, you're not really preventing anything. You're merely trying to keep a problem from getting worse. Thus, the healthcare and pharma industries' focus on too-far-downstream matters: the secondary and tertiary prevention we discussed in the previous chapter. Those are, to us, what Ben Franklin called "the pound of cure."

We are all constantly faced with a dilemma: the balancing act between a pleasurable short-term activity (Netflix from the comfy chair, a big sugary dessert, a cigarette, late nights out, etc.) compared to the far-off rewards of the behaviors that prevent something bad from occurring in the future. To some, the behaviors of prevention can seem like denial of pleasures, deprivation, and hard work. We prefer to see prevention as the acceptance of the potential realities of aging and the understanding that you can control as much as 75 percent of the way you age through lifestyle choices. (The remaining 25 percent is attributed to genes.)[48]

Our role at Activate Brain & Body is to motivate you to not only get started but also to demonstrate to you how amazingly rewarding this process will be in the present (activated brain, invigorated body, ignited spirit, and more), and to inspire you about how sensible that is in the long term.

Here are just a few of the ways that our ounce of prevention will be far preferable to many potential long-term outcomes:

Fall Prevention

We need to mention something many people wouldn't think about as being preventive healthcare. Since we are using the broadest, upstream definition of prevention, we need to go way upstream and talk about fall prevention.

Did you know that falls are the leading cause of accidental death in the senior population? One in four seniors falls every year—broken wrists, broken arms, and the dreaded broken hip. Two and one-half million seniors per year are treated for these injuries, and it costs over $60 billion in yearly healthcare costs.

According to the respected Mayo Clinic, fall prevention consists of things like reviewing your medications, wearing sensible shoes, removing home hazards, better lighting in your living space, and using assistive devices.[49] And while this is smart and useful advice, it's not upstream advice. Hidden within their recommendations is this: keep moving.

To us, that understated point is the start of where the vast majority of effort should be focused because you can actually train your brain and your body to better cope with the possibility and the after-effects of falling.

We believe the kind of fitness you will attain through The Cognitive Circuit™ and the related functional fitness exercises we offer are, in a very direct manner, the best way to prevent falls and their expensive consequences.

In addition to The Cognitive Circuit™, we have created a functional fitness workout called The FMR Circuit™ (flexibility, mobility, and relaxation).

Both The Cognitive Circuit™ and The FMR Circuit™ incorporate balance training that can help prevent some falls from happening in the first place. The circuits can give you the quick reflexes and muscle speed you need to recover from trips and occasional slips so that instead of falling on your wrist, elbow, shoulder, or hip, you can catch yourself before you fall.

An additional benefit of The FMR Circuit™ is relaxation and stress reduction, a critical element of better brain health. As we've learned, stress releases cortisol in your bloodstream, which is harmful to the creation of new brain cells. Less stress. Less cortisol. More brain cells.

Better Driving

Another area most would never think of as an upstream preventive healthcare benefit would be improved and safer driving skills. Can better brain and body health lead to safer driving? We believe it may do just that.

Driving is a source of independence, and this independence permits travel for fun, shopping, commuting to work, socializing with friends and family, and so much more. As a result, losing driving privileges is a significant turning point for people as they age. This loss of independence is life-changing, but can it be delayed?

Let's examine the facts. As the population ages, there are obviously many more aging drivers. Researchers have noted: "Older drivers, particularly those aged 75+, have higher crash death rates than middle-aged drivers (aged 35-54). Higher crash death rates among this age group are primarily due to increased vulnerability to injury in a crash."[50]

These statistics do not even begin to capture the extent of this growing issue since they do not include the uncounted and exponentially larger number of parking lot fender-benders, garage door scrapes, and minor dings that are the first signs of diminished driving skills.

The CDC conducted a landmark study examining the driving capabilities of older adults. They found that "Age-related declines in vision and cognitive functioning (ability to reason and remember), as well as physical changes, might affect some older adults' driving abilities."[51]

Specifically, people's driving skills begin to get worse as a result of diminished brain processing speed, which results in slower reaction times, decreased concentration and focus, poorer agility, and poorer vision. What we noticed is that these are the very things that the Activate Brain & Body programs address.

In the research and trial programs that led to The Cognitive Circuit™, some participants showed significant, measurable improvements in all of these areas. These findings led us to develop and integrate specific techniques that focus on brain and body training and have the potential to enable safer driving.

Fitness and Vision

The connection between the eyes and the brain is well documented. In fact, the optical nerve is actually an extension of your brain. Considering this, it seems sensible that actions to improve brain health, like building brain-derived neurotropic factor (BDNF) and new neural networks, would also benefit visual health. More and more optometrists are coming to this same conclusion, particularly following the guidance of an increasing number of studies.

One such study by the Veterans Optometry Partners of America explains how better fitness and brain health can impact visual health: "Exercise produces a chemical known as a brain-derived neurotrophic factor or BDNF. This chemical helps prevent age-related eye decline by reducing the amount of brain deterioration. Think of exercise as a maintenance program for the brain, if you will. Turn off the television, put down the phone, and get your blood flowing if you want to maintain good health, including great vision and eye health."[52]

With research showing the strong connection between brain and body health, how is Activate Brain & Body playing a role in reinventing fitness as upstream preventive healthcare?

Our model encourages people above age 45 to adopt lifestyles more conducive to better fitness, brain health, and longevity. This creates positive impacts on the numerous biometric measures of improved brain and body health.

 Our unique approach helps you create success through a well-researched system that:

- Motivates success by tapping into a deeper, more insightful understanding of behavior and fitness goals.

- Utilizes new technology to optimize brain and body fitness.

- Coaches individuals toward measurable results that matter to them.

- Understands the unique needs of individuals age 45 and up by helping them take charge of the way they age.

After following our program, you will be amazed by how medically boring your life can be. And you'll discover how much more satisfying it is NOT to be an ongoing revenue stream for the medical community.

If you don't want to drain your life savings and your retirement benefits on doctors, pills, and potentially massive medical expenses, stay active, engaged in life, and socially connected, and get fit. Being fit and active gives you the best chance to experience and enjoy the new vision of aging.

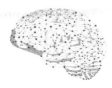

CHAPTER 11

A NEW VISION OF AGING

Aging is an extraordinary process where you become
the person you always should have been.
—DAVID BOWIE

In July 2021, Ms. Katherine Stilwell climbed to the top of Mount Monadnock in New Hampshire to celebrate her 90th birthday. According to her son-in-law, she is now trying to decide which mountain to climb for her 100th.[53]

Klaus Obermeyer, the founder of the Obermeyer sports clothing company, is still skiing at the age of 100. He jokes that "the first hundred years are behind me, now it's on to the next century...You have to keep exercising." He then doubles down on the importance of fitness, saying, "Your health should be your number one priority. Your body carries your brain. If your body is healthy, then your brain has a chance to be healthy, too."[54]

Ralph Jesseman is a recently "retired" corrections officer who says, "I chose life, and I'll be damned if I'm giving up. I'm 66, and I've known many 50-year-olds that are OLD!! People need to un-Velcro themselves from their couch and from self-limiting their existence." When we last checked in with Ralph, an avid high mountain hiker, he was averaging two White Mountain summits per week and guiding numerous friends and family in the process at a pace normally maintained by people half his age.

We could go on and on with stories of active agers like these three, who refuse to abide by the more traditional view of aging. While this attitude is a reality for some, there are, unfortunately, many more who lack this mindset.

One reason for this might be that most people drastically underestimate how much longer they're going to live. They buy into the generations-old standard that somewhere in your 60s is the appropriate time to slow down, relax, and retire. People who follow this path are unaware that you can, indeed, take charge and change the way you age.

Instead of actively aging, it seems too many people think they'll inevitably begin to fade in their late 60s or early 70s. With this mindset comes a feeling that they'll also be less useful and productive than when they were younger. We know this is far from true.

As we learned in chapter 2, trends show that making it to age 90 is quite probable, and age 100 is possible. As people live longer, they are starting to realize that the way you live your life, and especially the choices you make in your 40s and 50s, dictates how well you will age.

This brings us back to **the two most important things we've said throughout this book:**

1. You can, and should, take charge of the way you age.

2. It's never too early, or too late, to start.

Longevity Changes the Equation

When the average life expectancy was lower, it made sense to consider slowing down in your late 50s or early 60s. You could then enjoy a few years of relaxation and live off your retirement savings and Social Security, right? You had paid into these funds, and now it was time to get it back and enjoy life before your time was up.

But things have changed. People's thinking about age has shifted, and the economics around aging is also different. As people are starting to understand how to live longer, they're also starting to understand that the act of slowing down not only contributes to but can also accelerate the decline.

At Activate, all we can think of is how disappointing it is to see perfectly healthy and productive people decide they are done when their experience and wisdom still hold great value. Maybe it's not an entirely conscious decision. Some time off sounds great, right? But entering a retirement mindset too early can result in people not challenging their minds or their bodies. They begin to willingly slide down that curve of aging, and that seems to us to be a terrible mistake, driven by the wrong attitude. More people need to open themselves to the new paradigm of aging and recognize that physical and mental challenges keep them healthy and engaged.

This is uniquely possible in today's world, where experience and wisdom are recognized as invaluable. Even when the average age of a Google or Facebook employee is 29, and ageism is increasingly rampant across corporate America, a small but growing segment of the business world and society is starting to realize that people in their 60s and 70s can be very valuable company and cultural assets.

For one, people with many years of experience do not struggle with challenges and problems the same way younger, inexperienced people do. They see things in the context of their many years of problem-solving and exposure to countless issues. They've developed an ability to see patterns and offer insights that people with fewer years and less experience cannot fathom.

Employers are starting to recognize the benefits of tapping into an aging workforce. According to research from the Milken Institute Center for the Future of Aging[55], older employees take fewer sick days, show stronger problem-solving skills, and are more likely to be highly satisfied at work than their younger colleagues.

What's your choice? Watching the waves on the beach as you grow old, awaiting the slow decline into senility and death, or taking a chance on you? At Activate Brain & Body, we're betting on you. We'll work with you to define future goals and help you accomplish them. This isn't the aging trajectory our parents and grandparents lived. It's a new paradigm that defies aging by activating both brain and body.

How About Rebooting Yourself?

While many of us may still dream of retirement's golden years, it may not be what you envision. A 2016 study[56] found that early retirement may be a risk factor for mortality. In fact, this study found that people who worked longer lived longer. These findings match other longitudinal studies that found correlations between retirement and poor health. Researchers speculate that the health benefits of working longer result from the positive effects of work environments that involve social interaction, movement, and a sense of purpose. Several studies have also linked retirement with loneliness and depression.[57]

But working long hours year after year is not the answer either, though some do choose to work at demanding careers well into their 70s and above. These are the folks who have stayed cognitively and physically active. Research shows that from mid-life onward, the sweet spot for health and longevity is working at a less intense pace and perhaps for fewer hours. It's a marathon, not a sprint; you can go much further if you slow your pace a bit as you age.

Work Longer. Live Longer.

Say you're able to retire with a secure pension or want to because you hate your job. You don't necessarily have to retire per se. Instead, find another vocation. Retrain and do something completely new. Retiring in the classic sense—to the beach, to the golf course, or to the sofa—is the quickest way to age fast, lose your sharpness, and slide down that path to oblivion. Finding a new opportunity where you can contribute will keep you young.

Not convinced? Here are some considerations:

Retire Too Soon

- You fade. If you stop moving and stop using your brain, you accelerate the downhill trajectory of aging.

- It's lonely. Your social connections dwindle. Loneliness is a key factor in depression and advanced aging.

- It's boring. You probably need something useful to do when the kids grow up and fly the coop.

Continue Work or New Vocation

- You gain a positive outlook. Satisfaction with life goes way up with age if you feel useful, productive, and fully engaged.

- You decrease financial worries. You'll have less anxiety about using up your retirement savings prematurely.

- You're not done yet. If you're not satisfied and at peace with your life's work, use your remaining years to do something more, something new, something productive and useful. Volunteer, teach, mentor, invent, write. Put all those remaining years to good use.

We should also focus beyond work and consider the many activities you can do with your newfound energy! Why not adventure travel, trekking, mountain biking, or surfing? You could even create a startup, begin consulting, or start coaching or mentoring. There are infinite numbers of ways to use your experience and time when you have the energy created by heightened brain and body fitness.

This is an overused and perhaps trite example, but it's worthy of repeating: Colonel Sanders did not start his Kentucky Fried Chicken business until he was in his 60s. While working to this age was practically a miracle in the late 1950s and 1960s, it is already fairly commonplace and is certain to become even more prevalent over the next generation.[58]

New Way to Age

So, yes, we are advocating for a new vision of aging. A vision where people are active, engaged in life to the fullest, and living productive, social, meaningful lives. These outcomes are possible by choosing to live a life that is healthy for both the brain and body.

At Activate Brain & Body, we call this new way of aging becoming The Activated Self™: a state you achieve when your brain and body function optimally.

Choosing to be fit and active gives you the best chance of living your best life for a long time. Attaining a new, higher level of fitness will make that time even more rewarding. You won't exhaust your life savings and retirement benefits on medical expenses or spend the last ten years of your life being driven from one doctor's office to another.

The much better alternative—and one that we at Activate Brain & Body believe is quite attainable—involves living a long, active, healthy life and then experiencing a brief amount of time in decline as we approach our last days. This is known as compressed morbidity, and it is a far more desirable goal for many people. With compressed morbidity, you avoid the long, slow, medically expensive, and emotionally distressing decline to death. Instead, you "live long, die fast."

So, now what?

You begin to take charge of the way you age and radically improve the trajectory of your aging. Choose to be part of the rapidly growing movement of actively aging people creating a new vision of aging. Get Activated!

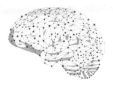

CHAPTER 12

GET ACTIVATED!

The secret of getting ahead is getting started.
—MARK TWAIN

Everyone, and we mean *everyone,* starts at the bottom with a single first step. We start as a neophyte, a newbie, an amateur, a greenhorn, a tenderfoot, an apprentice, a beginner.

Formula One race car drivers, airline pilots, Olympic athletes, elite endurance athletes, concert pianists, pro tennis players—all began as novices. They started at the beginning and attained great heights, but the most important action was the first step. As you start out, there is no need to feel anxious about starting a fitness routine. You begin your path to fitness, brain health, and longevity with a single first step.

The benefit of only having to take that single first step is that since it's small, there is a high probability you will succeed. You don't have to focus on the immensity of the task in front of you, which can be daunting. Instead, you merely have to take that one baby step. And we're here to help.

If losing weight is your big challenge, you only have to focus on losing that first pound or two. If trekking five miles up a hill is your challenge, you start by walking a mile on flat ground. If changing the trajectory of the way you age matters to you (and it should), start now because it's never too early or too late to begin. The steps you take now will be well worth it years down the road.

No matter how big a challenge, you can manage it by breaking it into a series of smaller challenges. Or, if you look at it from another perspective, the smaller, individual little steps add up to larger, manageable pieces, and over time, these add up to (surprise!) seriously big accomplishments.

For instance, committing to lose one pound per week adds up to losing 50 pounds in one year—a life-changing accomplishment. Increasing the distance you walk by only five percent per week means that by the end of six months, a one-mile walk becomes almost 3 1/2 miles. If you increase your walking distance by 10 percent per week, which is very possible, at the end of six months, you'll be walking 10 miles. Being able to do a 10-mile walk reflects a seriously good level of fitness, and that is a very achievable target for most people.

This same kind of thinking applies when you decide to take charge of the way you age. All you need to do is start with the first small steps combined with achievable goals, and the process has begun.

Getting Started

Taking the first steps may seem daunting, but that's why we're here. We can help you get started.

Here are a few signs that you're ready to Activate:

You've never participated in a fitness program or joined a gym. This is our specialty because we are not like traditional fitness clubs. At Activate Brain & Body, our coaches are extensively trained to work with beginners and those turned off by other options. You are never judged, and there is no competition with anyone else (except maybe a previous version of yourself). In fact, you will find comfort in knowing that many of our members are just like you in this regard.

You're looking for solutions to improve aging but have not found the answer.

You've noticed you're not as active as you once were and would like to recapture some youthful energy and stamina.

You're starting to notice you are becoming forgetful (i.e., where did you put the keys, why did you walk into a room, etc.). Important dates sometimes take a while to recall, or you forget where and when you have to be somewhere.

You often feel overwhelmed and overstressed with tasks.

You want to take charge of your future and take preventative action.

You want to become healthier overall, and since you are focused on your health (losing weight, decreasing pain, improving strength), you also want to take the necessary steps to help build your brain.

Experiencing any or several of the above is part of the natural aging process and not anything to get overly stressed about. But as we've learned, the trajectory of aging can be slowed. You can delay, offset, stall, and hopefully prevent declines from becoming serious impediments to a long, happy, and healthy life span.

Even better, you now know a lot about the science of brain and body health and how the two are interconnected. You've learned that genetics may account for only 25 percent of the way you age and that the remaining 75 percent is up to you.

You get it, and you're ready to get started, but what should you do first?

Preparing for Your Fitness Journey

There are a few things you can do as part of your fitness journey, and we will repeat them here:

- First, schedule a visit with a healthcare professional and get a physical. This guarantees that you're ready to get started. If any restrictions are identified, these can easily be incorporated into your program.

- Next, if you smoke, quit—right now. We cannot emphasize this enough. The perfect time to do it is when you begin a program for brain health.

- If you're not currently active, take baby steps by adding movement into your day. Start with walking. It doesn't matter where—outside, inside on a treadmill, at the mall, or at your current gym. You can enlist a friend or go it alone, but go ahead and go for a walk.

- If you are currently active, mix it up. Change routes or add intensity to a treadmill workout by intermittently changing the incline or by alternating between high and low intensity.

- Add some cognitive challenges to your day. For example, try saying the alphabet backward while walking. When that's no longer challenging, count back from 100 by subtracting three from each number.

- Get a fitness tracker. Fitbit, Garmin, Polar, and Apple Watch are just some of the available options that can help track your progress towards becoming a better you. (If you're in Cincinnati and working out with us, we'll provide a MyZone belt to new members because it is an integral part of our membership and the coaching process.)

Getting Started in the Cincinnati Area

Please make an appointment to meet with one of our coaches, all certified brain health trainers. Our experienced coaches are ready to help you and have additional accredited certifications in personal training, functional training, and group training.

They have years of experience coaching people at all levels and know how to help clients set and reach their goals. They know that *personal* fitness does not come with a one-size-fits-all approach. Our coaches take the time to learn what's important to you and create customized plans to help you achieve your goals.

You now have the information and tools to get started. It's time to take the next step on the journey to living your longest and healthiest life.

Get Smarter About Brain Health

For more about brain health and the vital role of exercise, we think you'll enjoy these books:

Spark: The Revolutionary New Science of Exercise and the Brain (Ratey and Hagerman, 2008). A groundbreaking investigation into the transformative effects of exercise on the brain from a renowned psychiatrist.

Keep Sharp: Build A Better Brain At Any Age (Gupta, 2021). A science-driven guide to protecting your mind from decline by neurosurgeon and CNN chief medical correspondent Sanjay Gupta.

The MIND Diet: A Scientific Approach to Enhancing Brain Function and Helping Prevent Alzheimer's and Dementia (Moon, 2016). A guide to a new breakthrough diet that's shown to keep your mind sharp as you age.

Secrets of Aging Well: Get Outside (Martin Pazzani, Activate Brain & Body Chairman and Co-Founder, and avid hiker, 2020). Why hiking may be the proverbial 'fountain of youth' and remarkable brain fitness activity. Be Healthier, Recharge Your Brain, Prevent Burnout, Find More Joy, and Maybe Live to be 100.

Lifespan: Why We Age and Why We Don't Have To (Sinclair, 2020). An authority on genetics and longevity, Sinclair reveals a bold new theory for why we age. As he writes: "Aging is a disease, and that disease is treatable."

The First 20 Minutes: The Surprising Science of How We Can Exercise Better, Train Smarter, and Live Longer (Reynolds, 2013). A *New York Times* bestseller that explains how groundbreaking scientific discoveries can help each of us achieve our personal best.

The SharpBrains Guide to Brain Fitness (Fernandez, 2013). How to Optimize Brain Health and Performance at Any Age.

READY TO START YOUR JOURNEY? READY TO GET ACTIVATED?

If you are in the Cincinnati area, you can schedule an appointment with one of our certified brain health trainers by calling (513) 793-2724. Make sure you mention our EXCLUSIVE 4-week program, and we'll get you started.

Keep up to date on brain health news and Activate Brain & Body locations by following us on Facebook here: https://www.facebook.com/ActivateCincinnati

Let's stay connected. Sign up for our newsletter to find out the latest brain health discoveries and tips: ActivateBrainAndBody.com/newsletter.

We look forward to helping you on your journey to a better brain and better body. Remember, it's never too soon, and it's never too late to take charge of the way you age.

NEW MEMBER EXCLUSIVE OFFER: 4-WEEK PROGRAM
$349 program for ONLY $99

Your personalized program includes:
- 16 total workouts
  - » 3 sessions per week of The Cognitive Circuit™. Our proprietary workout is designed to activate your brain and invigorate your body.
  - » 1 session per week of The FMR Circuit™. Our proprietary workout is designed to improve flexibility and mobility while reducing stress
- 28 days of brain-based nutrition guidance
- 2 comprehensive assessments (one at the start to establish a baseline and one at the end of your 4-week program to measure progress)

This program is valued at $349 and is yours for ONLY $99.

Offer valid for new Members only and expires June 30, 2022.

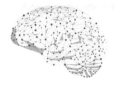

THANK YOU

We appreciate your interest in Activate Brain & Body and thank you for taking the time to read this book.

As we stated in the preface, our company was founded by a group of people united around a mission: **to radically improve the trajectory of aging and to operationalize what we have learned about creating brain fitness.** This book contains much of what we've learned and why it is so relevant to a world with a rapidly aging population increasingly concerned about the way they age, their healthcare costs, and the quality of their life spans.

We believe we can help you to live a happier, healthier, and longer life. Our approach can give you the independence to do whatever you desire, whether that's continuing to work productively, enjoying sports or travel, spending time with great-grandchildren, and so on.

We believe we can also reduce your long-term healthcare costs by slowing, minimizing, or preventing the conditions that shorten your health span: cognitive decline, dementia, metabolic syndrome, and more. Our approach empowers you to ignore and overcome the indignities of aging and remain active, sharp, independent, and vital.

And, of course, the best news of all is that when you focus on building better brain health, you also build a much better body. That's why we say "Put Your Brain First"—because your body will follow.

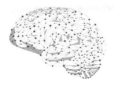

GLOSSARY

A brain health center is a new concept, which means it also uses new terms and phrases. While most are not new, they may not be familiar concepts. Since we use these terms throughout the book, we thought a glossary would be helpful.

Alzheimer's Disease
Alzheimer's disease, the most common cause of dementia, is a progressive neurologic disorder that causes the brain to shrink (atrophy) and brain cells to die.

BDNF / Brain-Derived Neurotrophic Factor
BDNF, often referred to as "Miracle-Gro for the brain," is a growth factor protein that improves the function of neurons (brain cells), encourages new neurons to grow, and protects neurons from cell death. Exercise has been shown to increase the levels of BDNF in the hippocampus, the area of the brain associated with memory.

The Cognitive Circuit™

The Cognitive Circuit™ is the Activate Brain & Body proprietary workout that consists of a combination of activities that include cognitive challenges during or following physical exercise once the heart rate has been elevated to stimulate the production of BDNF. The specific activities performed within The Cognitive Circuit™ target each member's individual goals and fitness level.

Cognitive Training

Cognitive training is comprised of activities designed to stimulate the brain. This is similar to how physical training is comprised of activities that exercise the body and improve physical fitness.

Cognitive Reserve

Cognitive reserve is a concept developed by researchers in the 1990s to explain how some people cope better than others with the same amount of damage to the brain. The cognitive reserve theory proposes that these individuals have stronger and more flexible neural networks that can compensate for damage. Modifiable lifestyle behaviors that support neurogenesis and positive neuroplasticity have been shown to be the most powerful contributors to cognitive reserve, and it is these behaviors that form the foundation of the Activate program.

Dementia

Dementia is the loss of cognitive function. Once healthy neurons in the brain stop working, lose connections with other brain cells, and die. Dementia is more common as people grow older, but it is not a normal part of aging.

Dual Tasking

Dual tasking, a cornerstone of The Cognitive Circuit™, combines aerobic exercise (Task #1) to generate neurons with cognitive challenges (Task #2) to build new neuropathways that can create cognitive reserve. Research suggests that in addition to being more efficient, dual tasking is more effective than single-tasking, particularly for improving memory and attention.

Functional Fitness

Functional fitness exercises train your muscles to work together and prepare you for daily tasks by simulating common movements you might do at home, at work, or in sports. For example, a squat is a functional exercise because it trains the muscles used when you rise up and down from a chair or when you pick up objects from the floor.

Health Span

The part of a person's life during which they are generally in good health. Currently, there is an average gap of 20 plus years between health span (healthy years) and life span (total years). Activate Brain & Body has made enhancing and extending health span one of our goals.

Longevity Economy

The total portion of economic activity that serves the needs of Americans over 50, including both products and services. It also includes the rapidly growing economic contributions of older adults. AARP reports in The Longevity Economy® Outlook[59] that the 50-plus age cohort contributes $8.3 trillion to the U.S. economy each year, or 40 percent of the U.S. gross domestic product (GDP).

Neural Pathways

Neural pathways are a series of connected nerves along which electrical impulses travel in the body. These pathways connect two or more different neurons, facilitating communication between them.

Neurogenesis

Every day, through a process called neurogenesis, thousands of new neurons (brain cells) are produced in the adult hippocampus, which is the brain structure central to memory and learning. Neurogenesis is crucial when an embryo is developing, but it continues to impact certain brain regions after birth and throughout our life span.

Neuroplasticity

Neuroplasticity refers to the flow of neurons, their connection to networks, and the strengthening or weakening of those networks. Positive neuroplasticity (strengthening) has been shown to occur with many modifiable lifestyle behaviors, such as physical activity and cognitive stimulation.

Physical Reserve

The capability of an organ to carry out its activity under stress is known as physical reserve. A healthy individual is considered to attain their peak physical reserve around the age of 25, after which the reserve starts to decline as the individual ages. However, physical reserve can be replenished through activities such as aerobic exercise and strength training, and it really doesn't matter at what age you start.

Quantified Self

Quantified self refers to the cultural phenomenon of using technology to measure, track, and compare activities related to one's own performance and often in comparison to others.

The Activated Self™

The Activate Self™ is when your brain and body function optimally.

Upstream Preventive Healthcare

Our focus on upstream preventive healthcare means that you have an opportunity to take charge of the way you age. You can potentially prevent a condition from ever existing—upstream to when a condition has already surfaced.

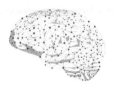

ABOUT THE AUTHORS

This book is a collaboration from the founding partners at Activate Brain & Body. The principle collaborators are:

Rexford Bevis, Chief Financial Officer
Mike Gelfgot, Chief Operating Officer
Alison Kal, Chief Marketing Officer
Adam Ortman, Chief Coaching Officer
Martin Pazzani, Chairman and Co-Founder
John Spence, CEO & President
Marie Stoner, Chief Science Officer and Co-Founder

For more information about the authors and the company, please visit www.activatebrainandbody.com.

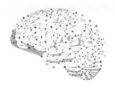

ENDNOTES

1. Ridder, M., 2021. *Size of the anti-aging market worldwide 2020 | Statista*. [online] Statista. Available at: <https://www.statista.com/statistics/509679/value-of-the-global-anti-aging-market/> [Accessed 1 September 2021].

2. Gough, C., 2021. *Topic: Health & Fitness Clubs*. [online] Statista. Available at: <https://www.statista.com/topics/1141/health-and-fitness-clubs/#:~:text=The%20market%20size%20of%20the,Fitness%20and%20Life%20Time%20Fitness> [Accessed 1 September 2021].

3. Booth, F., Roberts, C. and Laye, M., 2021. Lack of Exercise Is a Major Cause of Chronic Diseases.

4. U.demog.berkeley.edu. 2021. *Life expectancy in the USA, 1900-98*. [online] Available at: <https://u.demog.berkeley.edu/~andrew/1918/figure2.html> [Accessed 1 September 2021].

5. The United States Census Bureau, 2018. *The Population 65 Years and Older in the United States: 2016*. U.S. Department of Commerce, p.1.

6. Shibata, M., 2019. With increased lifespans, elders are living thousands of days longer. That's very good news for the global economy. *BBC*, [online] p.1. Available at: <https://www.bbc.com/worklife/article/20190930-the-untapped-potential-of-the-longevity-economy> [Accessed 1 September 2021].

7. CBS, 2014. *Can your mental attitude reverse the effects of aging?* [video] Available at: <https://www.youtube.com/watch?v=DAZRHWl6UdE> [Accessed 1 September 2021].

8. Levy, B., Slade, M., Kunkel, S. and Kasl, S., 2002. Longevity increased by positive self-perceptions of aging. *Journal of Personality and Social Psychology*, [online] 83(2), pp.261-270. Available at: <https://www.apa.org/pubs/journals/releases/psp-832261.pdf> [Accessed 1 September 2021].

9. Abbott, E., 2019. *Ten percent of all healthcare spending in the U.S. goes toward end-of-life care.* [online] WRVO Public Media. Available at: <https://www.wrvo.org/health/2019-09-30/ten-percent-of-all-healthcare-spending-in-the-u-s-goes-toward-end-of-life-care#stream/0> [Accessed 1 September 2021].

10. Csiszar, J., 2021. *Yahoo is now a part of Verizon Media.* [online] Yahoo.com. Available at: <https://www.yahoo.com/now/average-retirement-age-every-state-190000202.html?> [Accessed 1 September 2021].

11. Knight, R. and McDaniel, C., 2012. Do those who retire early live longer? *BBC*, [online] Available at: <https://www.bbc.com/news/magazine-18952037> [Accessed 1 September 2021].

12. Tucker A, Stern, Y. *Cognitive Reserve in Aging.* Current Alzheimer Research (2011).

13. Fowler, Danielle. 2019. May 17. https://finance.yahoo. com/news/fast-walkers-longer-lifeexpectancy-120210928. html?ncid=facebook_yfsocialfa_wje3x23a50w&utm_ content=bufferbf522&utm_medium=social&utm_ source=facebook. com&utm_campaign=yahoofinance&fbclid =IwAR3XKpz5pO86Ke1_VA_sXe-S58DO3VToUMumQ64T-sEdfSNfhYizntTRb6X4

14. Verghese, J., Lipton, R., Katz, M., Hall, C., Derby, C., Kuslansky, G., Ambrose, A., Sliwinski, M. and Buschke, H., 2003. Leisure Activities and the Risk of Dementia. *New England Journal of Medicine,* [online] 349(13), pp.1290-1292. Available at: <https://www.nejm.org/doi/full/10.1056/NEJMoa022252>.

15. Mayo Clinic. 2021. *Mediterranean diet for heart health.* [online] Available at: <https://www.mayoclinic.org/healthy-lifestyle/ nutrition-and-healthy-eating/in-depth/mediterranean-diet/art-20047801> [Accessed 1 September 2021].

16. Medicalnewstoday.com. 2019. *Deep sleep: Stages and how much you need.* [online] Available at: <https://www.medicalnewsto-day.com/articles/325363?fbclid=IwAR08Omnxqu5589GumKS jOj2fyK3IKfOeFgB49kbWFehm891bM9ChNmCJjHo#stage-t wo> [Accessed 1 September 2021].

17. En.wikipedia.org. 2021. *Glymphatic system - Wikipedia.* [online] Available at: <https://en.wikipedia.org/wiki/Glymphatic_sys-tem> [Accessed 1 September 2021].

18. Booth, F., Roberts, C. and Laye, M., 2021. Lack of Exercise Is a Major Cause of Chronic Diseases. [online] https://www.ncbi.nlm.nih.gov/pmc/articles/PMC4241367/. Available at: <https://www.ncbi.nlm.nih.gov/pmc/articles/PMC4241367/> [Accessed 20 September 2021].

19. Publication. *Wearable Technology Market - Global Forecast to 2026.* MarketsandMarkets, April 1, 2021. https://www.asdreports.com/market-research-report-577503/wearable-technology-market-global-forecast.

20. Fnfresearch.com. 2021. Global Telehealth Market Size & Share Projected to Rise to USD 475.50 Billion By 2026. June 2021

21. Lynn, John. *Decline of Health and Fitness Tracker Usage.* May 21, 2014. https://www.healthcareittoday.com/2014/05/21/decline-of-health-and-fitness-tracker-usage/.

22. Anderson-Hanley, C., Arciero, P., Brickman, A., Nimon, J., Okuma, N., Westen, S., Merz, M., Pence, B., Woods, J., Kramer, A. and Zimmerman, E., 2012. Exergaming and Older Adult Cognition. *American Journal of Preventive Medicine,* [online] 42(2), pp.109-119. Available at: <https://s3.amazonaws.com/docs.ifholdings.com/CyberCycleStudy.pdf>.

23. BrainHQ from Posit Science. 2021. *Science Team & Research Partners - BrainHQ from Posit Science.* [online] Available at: <https://www.brainhq.com/world-class-science/science-team> [Accessed 1 September 2021].

24. Staff, A., 2017. *Study finds group exercise reduces stress more than solo workouts do - The DO*. [online] The DO. Available at: <https://thedo.osteopathic.org/2017/10/study-finds-group-exercise-reduces-stress-solo-workouts/> [Accessed 1 September 2021].

25. Medicine, N., 2021. *4 Habits of "SuperAgers"*. [online] Northwestern Medicine. Available at: <https://www.nm.org/healthbeat/healthy-tips/4-habits-super-agers> [Accessed 1 September 2021].

26. CDRG. 2021. *Inflammation | CDRG*. [online] Available at: <https://www.cdrg.org/chronic-diseases/inflammation/?gclid=CjwKCAjwybyJBhBwEiwAvz4G78cvp6m-oQm7o-3QIH8ZbHQLcYvZHwnx9WPTHJD4oTShofcofx2cJFRo-C2yYQAvD_BwE> [Accessed 1 September 2021].

27. Vishnevsky, J., 2020. Thinking of Hiring a Personal Trainer? Here's What You Should Know. [online] Redbook. Available at: <https://www.redbookmag.com/body/health-fitness/g33457819/working-with-personal-trainer/#:~:text=Working%20out%20with%20a%20personal,...go%20for%20it!> [Accessed 1 September 2021].

28. NICM, Western Sydney University. 2017. "Exercise Increases Brain Size, New Research Finds." November 13. https://www.sciencedaily.com/releases/2017/11/171113195024.htm.

29. Cleveland Clinic Newsroom. 2019. "Can Obesity Impact the Size of Your Brain?" March 2019. https://newsroom.clevelandclinic.org/2019/03/12/can-obesityimpact-the-size-of-your-brain/.

30. Ballantyne, Coco. 2009. "Does Exercise Really Make You Healthier?" January 2. https://www.scientificamerican.com/article/does-exercisereally-make/.

31. Jeurissen, Al. 2003. "The effects of physical exercise on the immune system." PubMed.gov, July 12.

32. Center For Disease Control and Prevention. 2020. National Center for Health Statistics. https://www.cdc.gov/nchs/fastats/leading-causes-of-death.htm

33. Martin, Stephen. 2009. "NCBI." NCBI. October 1. https://www.ncbi.nlm.nih.gov/pmc/articles/PMC2803113/.

34. Martin, Stephen. 2009. "NCBI." NCBI. October 1. https://www.ncbi.nlm.nih.gov/pmc/articles/PMC2803113/.

35. Crouch, Michelle. 2019. "To Live Longer, Exercise Daily." January 8. https://www.aarp.org/health/healthy-living/info-2019/exerciselongevity-wellness-benefits.html

36. Sifferlin, Alexandra. 2018. Time.com. February 20. https://time.com/5166564/physical-exercise-can-increase-lifespan/.

37. Lemar, Marissa Cruz. 2019. "Never Exercised in Your Life? It's Not Too Late to Start — and Benefit." October 21.

38. 2019. Diabetes and Obesity. January 15. https://www.diabetes.co.uk/diabetes-and-obesity.html

39. Sampath Kumar, A., Maiya, A., Shastry, B., Vaishali, K., Ravishankar, N., Hazari, A., Gundmi, S. and Jadhav, R., 2021. Exercise and insulin resistance in type 2 diabetes mellitus: A systematic review and meta-analysis.

40. American Cancer Society. 2016. "Exercise Linked With Lower Risk of 13 Types of Cancer." May 17. https://www.cancer.org/latest-news/exerciselinked-with-lower-risk-of-13-types-of-cancer.html.

41. Mayo Clinic. 2019. "Your secret weapon during cancer treatment? Exercise!" June 11. https://www.mayoclinic.org/diseases-conditions/cancer/in-depth/secret-weapon-during-cancer-treatment-exercise/art-20457584.

42. Mayo Clinic. 2014. "Slowing or Reversing Muscle Loss." April 10. https://www.mayoclinic.org/medical-professionals/physical-medicinerehabilitation/news/slowing-or-reversing-muscle-loss/mac-20431104.

43. Statista. 2021. Gym memberships in the U.S. 2000-2017 | Statista.

44. Gym memberships in the U.S. 2000-2017 | Statista, 2021)

45. Cms.gov. 2021. NHE Fact Sheet | CMS. [online] Available at: <https://www.cms.gov/Research-Statistics-Data-and-Systems/Statistics-Trends-and-Reports/NationalHealthExpendData/NHE-Fact-Sheet> [Accessed 18 October 2021].

46. Stephen Schondelmeyer, Leigh Purvis. 2018. AARP. September. https://www.aarp.org/content/dam/aarp/ppi/2018/09/trends-inretail-prices-of-brand-name-prescription-drugs-year-end-update.pdf

47. Psychology Today. 2021. *The Problem With Prevention*. [online] Available at: <https://www.psychologytoday.com/us/blog/happiness-in-world/201006/the-problem-prevention> [Accessed 18 October 2021].

48. Lemar, Marissa Cruz. 2019. "Never Exercised in Your Life? It's Not Too Late to Start—and Benefit." October 21. https://www.washingtonpost.com/lifestyle/wellness/never-exercisedin-your-life-its-not-too-late-to-start--and-benefit/2019/10/18/fd9b9342-f037-11e9-b648-76bcf86eb67e_story.html?fbclid=IwAR3-YLwRFE8BbU0m9LqxIE9A-syrCncEC-Mz5tB4UN5lgSRy1o6zpfi23zMg

49. Mayo Clinic. 2021. *Fall prevention: Simple tips to prevent falls*. [online] Available at: <https://www.mayoclinic.org/healthy-lifestyle/healthy-aging/in-depth/fall-prevention/art-20047358> [Accessed 18 October 2021].

50. Cdc.gov. 2021. *Older Adult Drivers | Motor Vehicle Safety | CDC Injury Center*. [online] Available at: <https://www.cdc.gov/transportationsafety/older_adult_drivers/index.html> [Accessed 18 October 2021].

51. Centers for Disease Control and Prevention. 2021. *Older Driver Safety*. [online] Available at: <https://www.cdc.gov/features/older-driver-safety/index.html> [Accessed 18 October 2021].

52. Veterans Optometry Partners of America. 2021. *Will Exercising Improve My Eyesight?*. [online] Available at: <https://vopa.org/will-exercising-improve-my-eyesight/> [Accessed 18 October 2021].

53. https://www.wmur.com. 2021. *Woman climbs Mount Monadnock for her 90th birthday*. [online] Available at: <https://www.wmur.com/article/woman-climbs-mount-monadnock-for-her-90th-birthday/36962098>

54. Averill, Graham. 2020. Outside Online. January 16. https://www.outsideonline.com/2407738/100-year-old-klausobermey-er-skier.

55. Irving, Paul. "Aging Populations: A Blessing For Business | Milken Institute". *Milkeninstitute.Org*, 2021. https://milkeninsti-tute.org/article/aging-populations-blessing-business.

56. LaPonsie, Maryalene. 2018. "Could an Early Retirement Help You Live Longer?" June 21. https://money.usnews.com/money/retirement/articles/2018-06-21/could-an-early-retirement-help-you-live-longer

57. LaPonsie, Maryalene. 2018. "Could an Early Retirement Help You Live Longer?" June 21. https://money.usnews.com/money/retirement/articles/2018-06-21/could-an-early-retirement-help-you-live-longer

58. Cheng, Michelle & Kopf, Dan. 2019. "The Number of Americans Working in Their 70s is Skyrocketing." June 3. https://qz.com/work/1632602/the-number-of-americans-working-intheir-70s-is-skyrocketing/.

59. Leadership, AARP. "The Longevity Economy® Outlook". AARP, 2021. https://www.aarp.org/research/topics/economics/info-2019/longevity-economy-outlook.html.

Made in the USA
Monee, IL
28 December 2021

87219663R00079